DIRTY, LAZY, KETO

DIRTY, LAZY, KETO

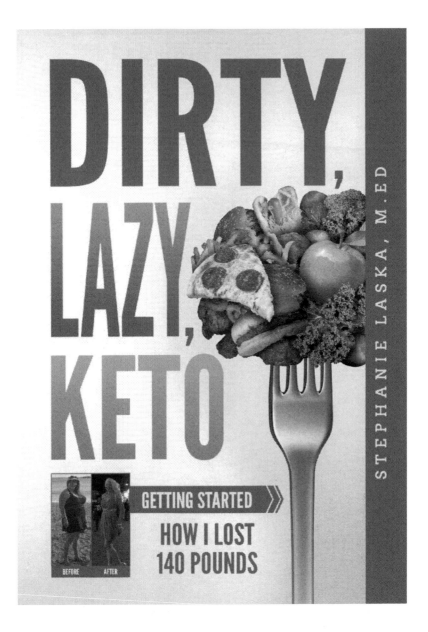

STEPHANIE LASKA, M.ED

BEFORE AFTER

GETTING STARTED »

HOW I LOST 140 POUNDS

COPYRIGHT

You may contact the author:

http://DirtyLazyKeto.com
https://twitter.com/140lost
https://www.instagram.com/140lost/
https://www.facebook.com/140lost

Interact with the DIRTY, LAZY, KETO community by joining the author-led Facebook group:
https://www.facebook.com/groups/177473472816901

First Edition

Disclaimer: This book is not written by a medical professional and is not intended to be a substitute for medical advice. This is for entertainment purposes only. Please consult your health care provider for medical advice and treatment.

Credits: Edited by William Laska, Cover designed by Alerrandre

ISBN: 9781720029625

DEDICATION

I would like to dedicate DIRTY, LAZY, KETO to my Editor-in-Chief, best friend, and love of my life, William Laska. We walked, stumbled, and sometimes ran, every step of this journey together.

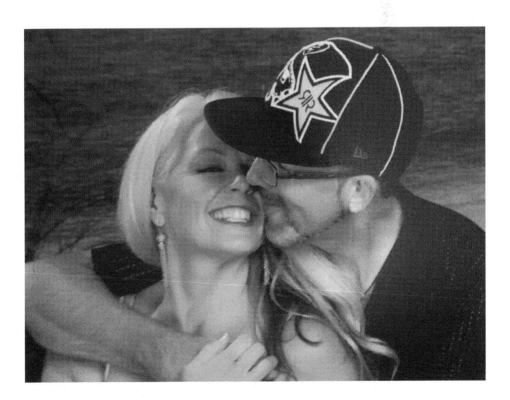

ACKNOWLEDGEMENTS

I would like to thank the many people that believe in me, my story, and my writing.

Thank you to the San Francisco Marathon for choosing me as a race Ambassador. By publishing my "inspirational story" with hopeful runners (even in a Groupon!), I was able to gain confidence as a writer and believe my story was worth sharing.

Thank you to the Big Sur International Marathon for sharing my "inspirational runner" story with thousands of athletes in your race guides. You helped me believe I had every right to be proud of finishing the marathon, even if I was finishing at the back of the pack.

Thank you to PowerBar® for choosing me to be a sponsored athlete for the New York City Marathon with the Clean Start Team. You taught me that with positivity and determination, I can and will overcome any obstacle in my path.

Thank you to Muscle & Fitness: HERS Magazine© for publishing my story. There is nothing like international exposure to help me overcome my embarrassment of dealing with health challenges while maintaining fitness.

Thank you to the Marathon Training Academy Podcast for sharing my articles about exercise and weight loss. You helped me find my writing voice as a writer.

Thank you to Bay to Breakers team for asking me to be their first race Ambassador. I hope to continue the message behind this amazing race that exercise can actually be fun!

Thank you to my longtime friend, dog walking companion, and sometimes editor, Dr. Tamara Sniezek, for endless conversations and humorous, empathetic debate about weight loss and all things related. She has encouraged me to "keep it real" and "be vulnerable" with my writing, so please thank her for my terrible jokes.

Thank you to author/podcast hosts: Gretchen Rubin, Elizabeth Craft, Sarah Fain, Chris Guillebeau, Sheri Salata and Nancy Hala for inspiring me to be brave, take the plunge by sharing my story, and to live the bigger life.

Thank you to the thousands of members of my interactive Facebook Group: https://www.facebook.com/groups/177473472816901.

Your posts, questions, and support for one another motivated me to culminate my experience into this user-friendly guide. We are venturing into unchartered territory with Dirty, Lazy, Keto, and must help one another along every twist and turn.

TABLE OF CONTENTS

PREFACE

The ketogenic diet was originally developed in the 1920s as a therapeutic alternative to help pediatric patients control epileptic symptoms. The diet focused on consuming a higher amount of fats, an adequate amount of protein, and a low amount of carbohydrates.

The ketogenic diet was soon replaced with medication to help patients. It wasn't until publicity from American Film Director James S. Abrahams in the 1990s that the ketogenic diet regained momentum. After finding the ketogenic diet helped his severely epileptic son, this Hollywood celebrity used his connections to spread the word and help others. In addition to starting The Charlie Foundation, Abrahams directed *First Do No Harm©* starring Meryl Streep which explored the benefits of the ketogenic diet with regards to epilepsy.

The renewed interest in the ketogenic diet during the 1990s prompted thought leaders to explore it's benefits in other health arenas, namely, with regard to weight loss. Elements of the ketogenic diet are present in many pop culture diets you might be familiar with. The South Beach Diet™ or Atkins Diet™ might strike you as possessing some similarities.

In addition to weight loss, the ketogenic diet is currently being studied for its positive treatment effects in the arenas of:

*Neurology – Increasing clarity/focus, less migraines, better memory, Alzheimer's prevention, therapeutic treatment for autism, treatment for dementia

*Cardiology – Decreasing blood pressure, improving cholesterol profiles

*Oncology – Decreasing tumor cell viability through nutritional intervention

*Anti-Inflammatory effects – Reducing joint pain, arthritis, flare ups of psoriasis and other diseases affected by inflammation

*Reproductive Health - Stabilizing hormones, helping women with PCOS, increasing fertility

Dirty, Lazy, Keto was only inspired by the ketogenic diet. It is not a strict interpretation, and offers the reader a unique approach to weight loss. Dirty, Lazy, Keto offers the perspective only from the author, Stephanie Laska. You will see many of the traditional "rules" of keto broken throughout the book.

BACKGROUND

W hen I first started following a DIRTY, LAZY, KETO eating plan, the only friend I had to ask for dieting advice was an alcoholic, Xanax fueled friend with an eating disorder. That being said, I didn't have much guidance! I didn't know the keto diet existed and had no idea that there were "others" out there eating in this way.

What I did know is that I was severely overweight – morbidly obese level III to be exact. I weighed close to 300 pounds. Even though (at the time) I didn't suffer from any obvious or immediate health problems, I knew if I didn't "do something" I would likely end up with diabetes or on an operating table having my stomach morphed into a ridiculous, unnatural shape. The fear of insulin shots or surgery (and fear of giving up Diet Coke® – isn't that a consequence of stomach surgery?) motivated me to consider all available options. **So how did I end up losing 140 pounds, about half of my total body weight?**

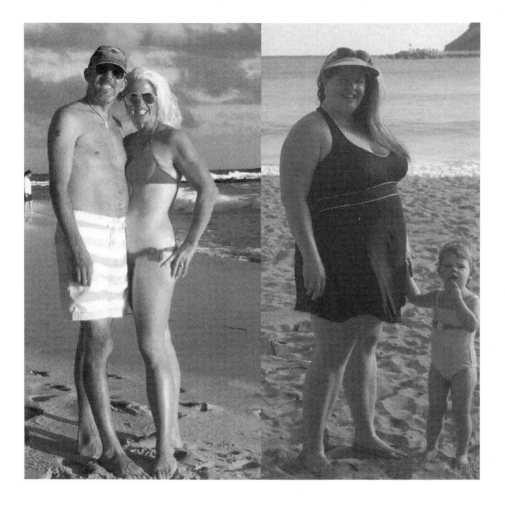

My pill-popping, wine swilling friend, crazy as she was, got me started down the path I would later groom into my current keto lifestyle. The purpose of this guide is not to memorialize my entire journey (that's for another book!), but rather, to get you started exactly where I finished. Why should you waste time in your journey making the same mistakes that I did? You don't want to hear all that drama (or do you)? Oh, dear reader, if you are interested in all of THOSE details then we are going to become long lost friends!

Before we move forward, I bet you want to clear up a couple of things...

WHAT DID YOUR FRIEND SAY? I bet you are curious! Now keep in mind that what she told me is not the secret behind DIRTY, LAZY, KETO. The sea did not part, and lights from heaven did not shine down upon me; there was not even a chorus of angels singing, "Hallelujah!" Quite the opposite -- this passing conversation was just the spark that ignited my metabolism in the right direction. Have you heard the saying about when the student is ready, the teacher shall appear? Well my teacher appeared as a middle-aged woman with a drinking problem!

I am happy to share with you the sad truth of what actually got me started. It's not glamorous, and actually it's downright embarrassing, but here goes: my friend shared that her formerly overweight husband was able to lose 40 pounds pretty quickly by eating a ton of grilled chicken while still drinking beer.

> *"SERIOUSLY!" I thought,*
> *"Losing weight while still drinking beer?*
> *NOW THAT'S MY KIND OF DIET."*

So, there it is. My friend went on to espouse the benefits of the Atkins Diet™. You might remember Dr. Atkins from the 1970s? Of course, you know what I'm talking about. No self-respecting overweight individual in America hasn't tried FREAKING EVERYTHING, right? I believed the Atkins program™ was about eating a lot of bacon, losing weight, and maybe having a heart attack, but other than that, I was actually pretty clueless. My training thus far, about losing weight, was limited to the calorie restriction model served up from years of attending Weight Watchers™ meetings[1] and listening to the rants from my ever weight-conscious grandmother.

I did glean *some information* from this Atkins™ conversation, though, that I would later find extremely helpful when launching my dieting

---

[1] *No disrespect to Weight Watchers™! Their program works for a lot of people, just not me.*

pilgrimage. Specifically, I learned that increasing protein and lowering carbohydrate intake would magically cause my metabolism to change and help me to lose weight. I didn't really care about all of the science behind how this worked as I was mainly focused on the weight loss (while enjoying eating grilled chicken and drinking beer) part of the story. That sounded like a win/win to me!

> *I got started. I added protein and healthy fats to my diet. I decreased carbohydrate intake. I lost some weight. THIS IS GOOD NEWS PEOPLE!*

I took that kernel of truth from Atkins™ and ran with it, morphing the rules AS I SAW FIT. Thus, I began the very long journey to where I stand today. It took about a year and a half to lose 140 pounds (roughly ten pounds a month), and I've kept it off for going on five years now. Over this time, with much trial and error, (LOTS of trial, LOTS of error), I've finally arrived at my own successful eating lifestyle that I have earned the right to call DIRTY, LAZY, KETO.

Please keep in mind that **this is my own version of keto**. I'm not following some website or existing plan touted by celebrities. This is the Stephanie Laska version, folks! What I'm about to share may challenge or even surprise you. So, before you get all "cray cray" on me, thinking of calling the keto police, I'd like to state the obvious: this here is my little book and I get to call the shots!

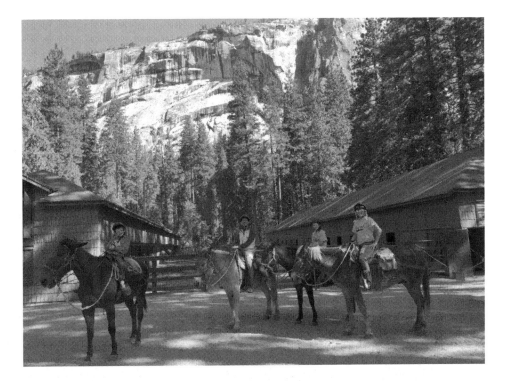

Finally, not over the weight limit!

For our last bit our housekeeping, I would like to address that in this mini-guide there is the potential for diet jargon to be used differently than what you have heard before. I may even introduce some new terms or (gasp!) use words differently than on other keto websites. This is my own version of dirty keto or lazy keto and even, "LAWD, help me!" my own version of the combined "dirty AND lazy" keto! *(Are those of you that are new to this keto business wondering what all of this shouting is about? Well, keto followers follow a variety of different paths and can sometimes be devout and EVANGELICAL about their beliefs. Therefore, I don't want semantics to prevent learning.)*

My goal with this mini-guide is to be the helpful friend to you that I never had. I want to give it to you straight and speak from experience. I come from a place of love, so forgive me if I offend or get it wrong occasionally! Truth be told, I welcome your feedback and hope to learn from you too. Life is a journey, my friends, not a destination.

> *My hope is that for the price of a movie ticket, you will spend roughly two hours reading through this mini-guide and leave armed with enough information to get started.*

I recently read a book about a meth addict and his sponsor (don't worry, I'm not headed down that path!). Something I took away from his memoir was the healing power of mentorship. The author talked about how becoming a sponsor to a person in need not only helped him "pay it forward" but surprisingly, also helped calm his own mind -- taking the focus off of himself. So perhaps, that is my motivation here. I feel I have been given a gift with my weight loss and now have a compulsion to help you, my dear reader.

> *I literally think about food, exercise, or weight loss with every waking moment of my day. I'm THAT kind of crazy.*

In conjunction with wanting you to achieve your dream of eating better and losing weight, it's also possible that I just want to stop the crazy voice in my head by putting my story down on paper. For all to see, here are my dirty, lazy keto beliefs, come what may!

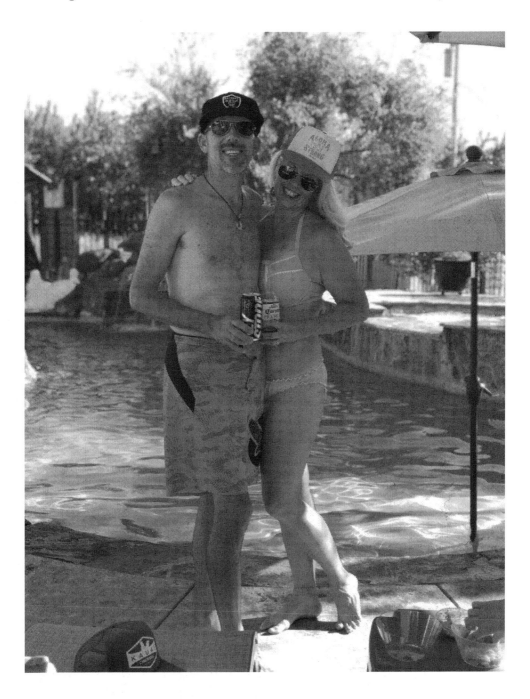

While I may have bit off more than I can swallow trying to cram this all in a short mini-guide, my goal is to get you started. Obviously, you've had a spurt of motivation (or curiosity) so let's capitalize on that and get you moving. No need to be long-winded here. I'm telling you it worked for me, and it sounds like you want to give it a try.

Will there be a lot of talk about the biology of weight loss? Um, no. That sounds really boring and plus, I'm not qualified. Although I am a former public-school teacher with a Master's Degree in Education, I will not be giving any science lessons here today, folks. Let's leave that up to the self-proclaimed keto experts, whomever they are! I'm not here to convince you to eat keto: lazy, dirty or otherwise. I just know this worked for me. I will give you enough soundbites to ward off your critical mother-in-law or insensitive coworker, but that's about it. DIRTY, LAZY, KETO is based largely on my own personal struggle to lose 140 pounds and keep the weight off for almost five years. Mic, dropped.

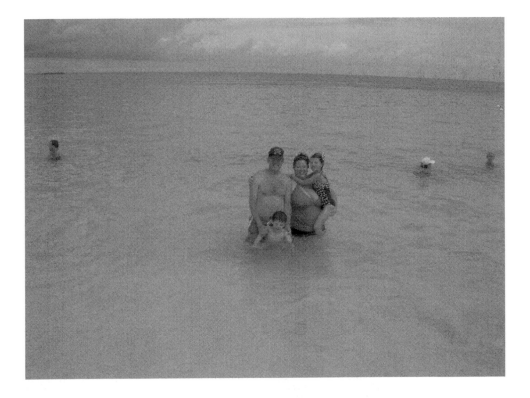

Ultimately, I want to provide you with real life inspiration and practical tips for getting started on a DIRTY, LAZY, KETO diet. Notice there won't be any discussion of the psychological components of weight loss – let's leave that HUGE topic for the next edition of <u>DIRTY, LAZY, KETO: The Reasons We Fail</u>, currently in the works for publication.

GOALS OF THIS MINI-GUIDE

L et's discuss the goals of this down and dirty mini-guide. By the end, you should be able to:

*Partner with your physician to set realistic goals based on your current health

*Understand the difference between a DIRTY, LAZY, KETO diet and a Ketogenic Diet

*Accurately read a nutrition label and count the net carbs per serving

*Confidently shop for ingredients that you need to be successful

*Stock your fridge and pantry with appropriate foods for cooking and snacking

*Prepare quick and easy meals, drinks, snacks, and desserts that are on plan

*Strategize ways to prevent dehydration

*Recognize and stop efforts at self-sabotage

*Have a long-term plan for healthy, sustainable weight loss

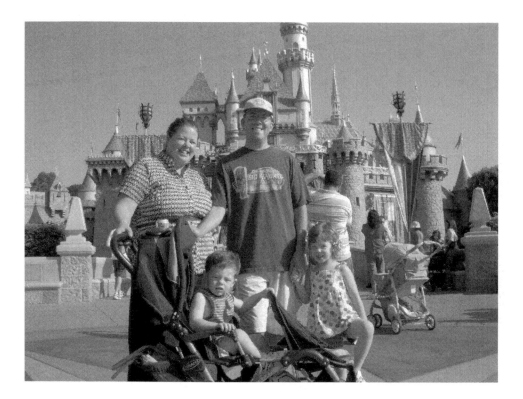

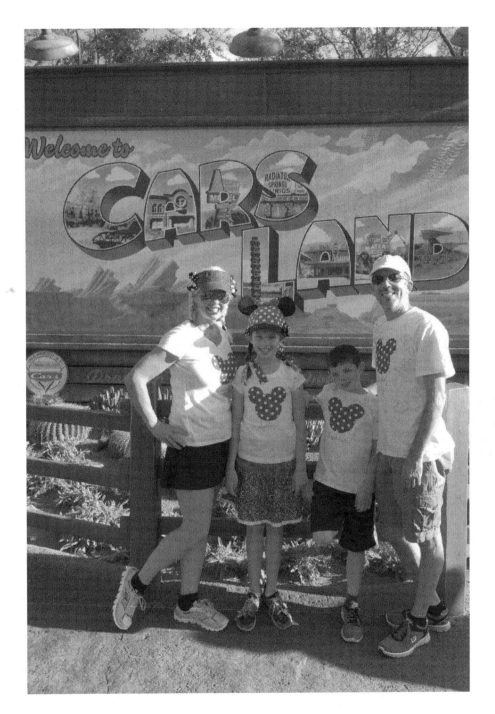

YOUR CURRENT HEALTH –

Talking to your Doctor, Setting Realistic Goals, and the Limitations of this Guide

I don't want to crush your excitement here about getting started, but before you begin, I urge you to check in with your physician. Yes, I hate going to the doctor too. The thought of some perky medical assistant getting all irritated because I want take an extra minute before stepping on the scale to remove my shoes and set down my purse is enough to raise my blood pressure AT LEAST ten points. If we are being honest here, I would prefer to strip down as bare as possible to get the lowest reading possible on that scale!

Checking in with your doctor is needed on many levels. You want to **get a "baseline"** of your current weight, blood pressure, cholesterol, A1Cs, etc., if not as a slap in the face to your current reality, than for you to use as a "I told you so" later on against keto skeptics.

> *When I was even modestly overweight, I always felt the doctors "blamed my obesity" for every health problem I sought help for. Whether this was actually substantiated or not, my avoidance of going to the doctor persisted until my weight ballooned to an unprecedented, all time high of close to 300 pounds. My avoidance was a hurdle I needed to overcome so I could team up with my health care provider to monitor my diet.*

You need to team up with your family physician when following a keto-inspired diet for your weight loss plan. I'm not a doctor, so I can't verify this program is appropriate for current health situation! Your health care provider can be a source of support and a sounding board. Think of your doctor as your personal consultant. Find a doctor that is educated about the merits of how you plan to lose weight. They are working for you as a paid consultant from your insurance (or pocketbook), so include them as a resource in this process.

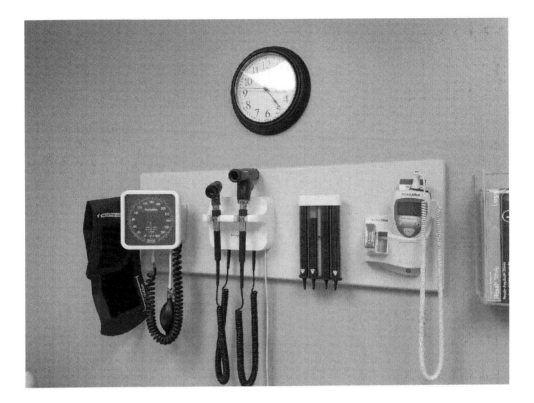

While your naked butt is sitting on the white paper covering the exam table, take a minute to really think about realistic goals. If you claim that your high school weight is your goal here, think again. It's time for a big-girl conversation (no pun intended, and sorry, gents) where a specific, measurable, achievable, realistic goal is needed to motivate you.

I had many goals starting out. Most seemed like far away dreams, but I want to share them with you in the interest of transparency. Here it goes! **I wanted to weigh less than my husband.** It's hard to feel good about yourself when your shirt size is triple that of your beau. We travel a lot together and I wanted to walk onto an airplane and be confident that the seat belt would close. When going out to eat, I hoped to sit at a booth, not just a table, without worrying if I could fit in the allotted space. If I went to the movies, I didn't want my thighs spilling over the arm rest onto my guy next to me. Oh man, I think I could go on and on here but I think you get the point.

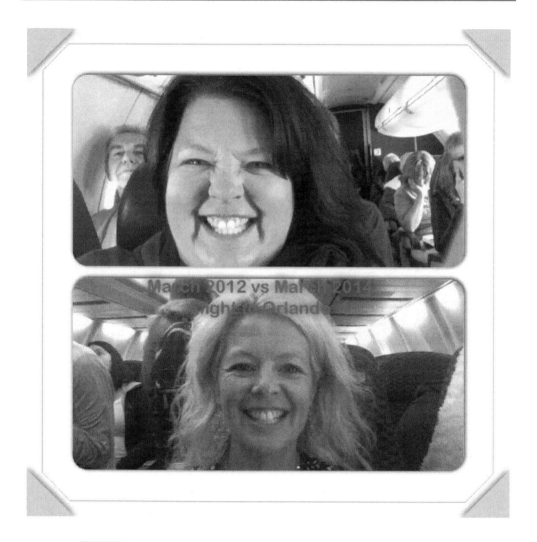

March 2012 vs March 2013 flight to Orlando

> *It's not just a number on the scale I sought after -- I wanted a life without embarrassment!*

Easily closing a seatbelt on an airplane never gets old.

LET'S GET THIS PARTY STARTED: WHAT IS A KETOGENIC DIET?

Without going into a bunch of science (snoooooooooze...), I want to give you enough info here to ward off questions from any crazy, critical co-workers or family skeptics. If you want to skip all of this background, go for it. Go to the next chapter, I dare you! Knowing all of this crap isn't going to make your weight come off any faster.

When I lost my weight, I had no idea what was happening. In fact, I was pretty mystified by the whole thing! None of it made sense to me at the time. I was like a little kid seeing what I could get away with. "Cheese? Ranch dressing? Sure, let's see what happens! OMG I still lost weight that week?

> *This is the WEIRDEST DIET EVER!"*
> *went through my mind every time I*
> *got on the scale.*

While I didn't want to ask too many questions (feeling like I would jinx the whole thing), I understand that you might be approaching this diet a bit more skeptically than I did. I learned all of this after the fact but am happy to share with you my armchair understanding of how it all works.

> *The focus of a ketogenic diet is to*
> *burn fat. That sounds good, right?*
> *Who wants to be fat? But you want*
> *me to eat lots of fat? This is so*
> *confusing!*

So how is this done? When the body is fed a diet that is low in carbohydrates, moderate in protein, and higher in fats, a new metabolic state is induced called "ketosis." Did I lose you there? Me too. You really don't need to know any of this, but I don't want you to be embarrassed when someone asks, "Why are you putting mayonnaise on that if you are on a diet?" etc. You can smartly reply, "Eating fats help put my body in ketosis!" (Now you sound legit.)

What is ketosis? Ketosis is a metabolic state where the liver produces "ketones" to be the main source of energy for the body. Ketones are like an alternative energy source for your body instead of glucose. When your body runs on ketones, your energy level is more constant without the "ups and downs" you experience on glucose.

For people like me who find themselves eating more whenever they get tired, this important distinction is a game changer. I have found that to avoid overeating, I need to eat a diet rich in healthy fats and lean protein, and lower in carbohydrates. This diet change helps me to maintain a consistent energy level. The fat and protein help stabilize my mood and energy throughout the day. I'm no longer searching in the kitchen or going through drive-thrus for food to help "lift me up".

This is the magical piece that helps me refrain from overeating and gaining weight (or maintaining an overweight body). Running my body on ketones also helps me only eat what my body really needs. I automatically reduce my caloric intake (WITHOUT COUNTING CALORIES!). This is how I lost weight.

IT'S A METABOLIC MIRACLE!

I would like to acknowledge the irony here of eating more fat to prevent getting fat or staying fat. I understand that is shocking, new information to many readers. To this day, I have to fight my impulses to NOT dip my artichoke into mayo. It just seems wrong! I was brought up in the 1980s where fat was blamed for almost everything, like obesity and heart disease.

> *I come from an era where SnackWell's™ cookies and Jazzercise™ were supposed to solve all of my weight problems.*

I'm here to tell you, as living proof, that we have been literally fed the wrong information! Fat is not evil. Fat is satiating! Furthermore, many of the fat-free products from our youth were supplemented with sugar to improve their taste. This is so wrong on many levels! **When the fat was removed in our foods and sugar was added, the remaining product was high in carbohydrates and not much else.** Eating a diet high in carbohydrates will cause your blood sugar to go haywire, just ask any diabetic.

Okay, this is getting complicated so let me step back. Think of your body like a car. You need to fuel your car to drive. When you go to the gas station, there are two types of fuel – economy gas and premium gas. Who knows what the difference is between the two? Don't we all just pick the cheapest gas and drive away? Both gas options get your car moving,

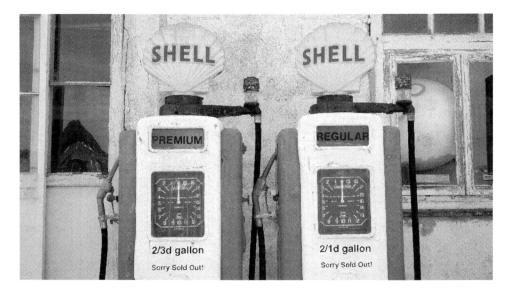

2/3d gallon

Sorry Sold Out!

2/1d gallon

Sorry Sold Out!

although one costs more and claims to be better for your engine. It's the same with your body. You have two ways to fuel your body's engine – either by consuming the cheap gas – glucose - or by making the premium gas – ketones. There! That makes sense, right?

What's wrong with the cheap gas – glucose? Everybody loves the glucose! Glucose is the body's immediate response to eating carbohydrates. Glucose is simply blood sugar; in fact, the Greek word for sweet is glucose. Whether you eat brown rice or a chocolate chip cookie, (despite one being obviously healthier than the other), both are quickly converted by your body into glucose. So not fair!

Glucose fuels your engine, true, but for many of us who are overweight, our engines process glucose differently (and perhaps inefficiently). When we eat a diet rich in carbohydrates, our body responds by converting that food into an energy source called glucose. The glucose swims around in our blood being led by the hormone insulin, fueling the various body systems. That sounds good, right? But like all good things, accepting glucose as a fuel source must be done in moderation. That's where the problems start. People like you and me tend to not eat carbs in moderation. Why is that?

Unlike the gas pump that shuts off when the tank is full, the body just keeps accepting more fuel. When we eat too many carbohydrates, too often, the body produces too much glucose and insulin, causing a backup. The body is smart and doesn't want to waste this energy. It converts the glucose to a longer lasting energy source: fat. (I know this is all super boring, and I myself am starting to fall asleep here. Let's get to the important part.)

Is this all our fault? Is the overproduction of glucose and insulin due to personal weakness or lack of will power? This is where I call BS. I'm so tired of the judgement and shame society places on the obese.

> *Metabolically, there is more at play here than just my own inability to put down the chips.*

I would like to propose a novel idea here. What if there is something wrong here with insulin, the hormone I mentioned earlier, in the obese? I'm going to go off on a tangent here but bear with me. There is a growing movement among researchers looking at insulin sensitivity and its role with weight loss. People who are more "sensitive" to their insulin are able to digest a higher level of carbohydrate (but not store excess glucose as fat). These are the skinny people we all hate that can eat anything. I am not one of those people, and I suspect neither are you.

Conversely, when you have a "weak" response to insulin (like me), you are called "insulin resistant". Even though my body is trying to tell me that I am full, I can't hear the voice. I just keep eating. There is no "off switch". Intellectually I know that over-eating is not good for me, but my body physically doesn't agree as I don't feel full. For example, I can get an extra-large popcorn at the movies and eat the entire tub *(and maybe part of the free refill if it's a long movie, just sayin')*. So why is my brain like this? That's just jacked up, people, and totally not fair.

Now I promised I wouldn't get "all scientifical" (yup, I made that one up!) so I'm going to wrap this up. At this time, there is no cure for being insulin resistant. It tends to worsen with age and can be caused by your genetics, family history of diabetes, or your ethnicity. IT'S SO NOT FAIR. We are not "normal" like the people who buy a small popcorn at the movies and feel full. I'm sorry.

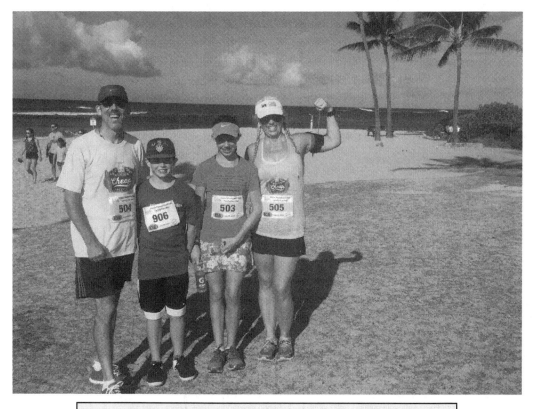

> ## No amount of will power or fat shaming will change your inner metabolism.

That being said, I have found that the DIRTY, LAZY, KETO diet helped me overcome these challenges with long-lasting results.

Are you convinced? Let's get started then. How about we take a look at the diet jargon that will be thrown around? This is like a secret handshake or gang sign (too far?) that will help you fit into your new keto tribe.

Glossary & Abbreviations

I would like to gently remind the reader that this is my own vocabulary list. I'll be using these terms fast and furiously, so I wanted to share with you my own definition of the terms, which may be different from what you have heard before.

Keto is simply a shortened word for ketogenic. It sounds a bit sexier and less medical, so let's go with that.

A **Ketogenic Diet** consists of eating a diet of foods that are: low carbohydrate, moderate in protein, and higher in fat with the goal of going into ketosis.

Ketosis occurs when the body burns ketones from the liver as the main energy source for the body (opposed to using glucose as the energy source derived from carbs.) Ketosis is often an indicator (but not a requirement) of weight loss.

Ketones are acids. Ketones occur when fat is breaking down. Ketones are often found in the blood and urine during weight loss.

Ketone Urine Testing Strips are just what you might expect. They are little strips of paper that when dipped in your urine will identify if your body has reached ketosis, or weight loss mode. I have never used a ketone urine testing strip, but I wanted to let you know about their availability. *I suspect just getting on the scale might be cheaper than buying these (and less messy), just sayin'.*

Calories are units of heat that a food provides to the body. There are no "good" or "bad" calories. You've got to let this one go, people! Calories are just a unit of measurement, like a cup or a gallon. Our bodies REQUIRE calories to survive. In keto-land, *we do not focus on calories*. The 80's are over, my friends, and counting calories and eating low-fat foods are a thing of the past.

Macronutrients or "**Macros**" There are three macronutrients: carbohydrates, proteins and fats. All macronutrients must be obtained through diet as the body cannot produce them. Macronutrients are necessary to fuel the body. There is no "good" macro or "bad" macro (though one of them is definitely my favorite – ahhh, carbo-liciousness). They all serve roles with nutrition and your health. All macros contain calories, though, but at different densities.

"Counting Macros" Instead of counting calories, many Keto dieters track their intake of macronutrients (protein, fats, and carbohydrates). You hear the phrase "counting macros" often in keto-land. Dieters might have a goal or a limit for each category, or a specific ratio to achieve each day with their eating choices. Many use apps or calculators to track their calculations. *I recognize that everyone is different, but I never used any gadgets. Just sayin'.* Now, I realize everyone is different, but I'm here to speak only on behalf of what worked for me. The only macro I ever counted was the carbohydrate.

Dirty Keto includes eating *whatever foods you choose* within your macro goals or limits (which are different for everyone). Dirty keto followers have a reputation (which may or may not be true) for including keto-friendly "junk food" into their diet (no judgment!). For example, if you want to eat a hot dog, then have at it, sister. This is your body and only you can decide what to eat or drink. Dirty keto means you play dirty and don't really follow any specific rules about your eating (other than the "big picture" of counting macro(s)). Artificial sweeteners and low carb substitutes are fair game. Dirty keto followers also don't limit their food or beverage choices, and might even be spotted drinking a Diet Coke® (*the horror!*).

Strict Keto has more "rules" about what you can and cannot eat. You might even call strict keto a "purist" style, where even the tiniest carb is called out and punished. (Sorry, did that sound judgmental?) For example, strict keto followers count even a splash of soy sauce or dollop of cream in their coffee when counting macros. Strict keto followers tend to frown upon artificial sweeteners, grain-based fillers, chemical additives, and sugars. Some might even count calories in addition to meeting macro goals and limits.

Lazy Keto followers only count carb intake, and do not track their consumption of fat grams or grams of protein. Please note that lazy keto does NOT mean you are lazy or unwilling to work hard for weight loss. This coined term refers to just one style of counting a single macro in keto – the carb -- and not a relaxed lifestyle or lack of energy.

Dirty and Lazy Keto dieters are a special breed that would like all the benefits of losing weight on a keto diet, but are not interested limiting food choices or counting every macro. Dirty and lazy keto followers only count the carbs they eat each day. They also incorporate artificial sweeteners (Diet soda or Splenda™ for example) and also eat packaged foods (protein bars, low-carb tortillas) as part of their diet. This is where I have ended up; I am the superhero of this category! Thus, the title of our book!

L.C.H.F. Diet that consists of eating **L**ow **C**arbohydrate, **H**igh **F**at foods (acronym) without the goal of ketosis. You may be totally shocked to learn that some skinny folks eat L.C.H.F. simply for reasons other than weight loss. Benefits of eating L.C.H.F. might include a reduction of inflammation, decreased joint pain, increased energy, or even to maintain weight loss.

Carbohydrates or "Carbs" are the sugars, starches, and fibers found in fruits, grains, vegetables and milk products. Foods high in carbs also include bread, pasta, beans, potatoes, rice and cereals. In general, packaged or processed foods in your pantry will be higher in carbs. Carbs contain 4 calories per gram. To further break down this category, I group carbs into two categories:

Slow Burning Carbs (my own made up term) have a higher fiber content and lower glycemic index. They are less likely to cause a spike in blood sugar. Slow burning carbs are more desirable in my opinion as they keep you feeling full longer and offer your body overall better health benefits than fast burning carbs. Examples would include non-starchy, high fiber vegetables like celery or broccoli. Slow burning carbs are your friends. They are more helpful than simple, fast burning carbs (in my opinion) at maintaining your blood sugar and preventing the vicious cycle of cravings.

Fast Burning Carbs (again, not a scientific phrase, just my own jargon) are simple sugars that quickly release glucose into the blood stream. These include processed carbohydrates such as breads, cereals, sugars, high sugar fruits and some starchy vegetables. Examples include candy, soda, pasta, potatoes, tortillas, or bananas. *This is the category of foods that cause me trouble!*

Net Carbs are the unit of measurement tracked in DIRTY, LAZY, KETO. When looking at a nutrition label, net carbs are calculated by subtracting the fiber grams and sugar alcohol grams from the listed amount of carbohydrates.

Protein has 4 calories per gram. Proteins take longer to digest since they are long chain amino acids. Protein is found in meats, dairy, eggs, soy, nuts, and seafood.

Fats are the densest form of energy, providing 9 calories per gram. Examples of fats are oils like olive oil or coconut oil; dairy foods like cream, butter, or cheese; eggs; nuts; avocados; fish like salmon; and in meats like dark meat chicken.

Fat Bombs are low carb, high fat desserts that are usually artificially sweetened.

Common Abbreviations in Social Media

SW – Starting Weight
CW – Current Weight
GW – Goal Weight
WOE – Way of Eating
WOL – Way of Living
NSV – Non-Scale Victory
SV – Scale Victory
IF – Intermittent Fasting
SF – Sugar-Free
LC – Low-Carb
HWC – Heavy Whipped Cream
SAD – Standard American Diet
RDA – Recommended Daily Allowance
SA – Sugar Alcohol
AS – Artificial Sweetener
BMI – Body Mass Index

WHAT THE HECK DO I EAT?

I just threw a lot of vocabulary at you, so take a breath and maybe even a break. Some of this might be new information for you to think about. I'm guessing you might even have strong opinions about what you just read. Good, great! That's what makes this plan so wonderful. You can tweak it to your heart's content. Personalize the hell out of it. Make it work for YOU.

> *I only want to share with you WHAT WORKED FOR ME. You can follow in my size 9.5 footsteps or blaze your own trail beside me.*

My only ask is that we stick together and support one another. Let's not judge each other for our personal tastes, budget, or life goals.

DIRTY, LAZY, KETO works best for me when I eat between 20-50 carbs/day. This is a big range, people! Some days (or weeks) I eat toward the lower end of the range (20), and some days at the higher end (50). Why is that? Was there some calculated nutritional plan in the works? NOPE! While I was losing 140 pounds, I did not have a strict plan. Real life was happening while I was trying to lose weight, and I needed some breathing room to account for roadblocks, challenges, and the dips in my motivation. Ultimately, by giving myself some wiggle room, I created a flexible environment where I could still be successful. I lost weight. It was freaking magical!

Everyone asks me, "HOW LONG DID IT TAKE?" What they are secretly wishing here is for a magic wand to melt away their fat instantaneously. I understand.

While I may have said all of this in the beginning, it doesn't hurt to remind you again, my dear reader, THAT THIS REALLY WORKS. I lost around ten pounds a month for about a year and a half. I lost 140 pounds total. Isn't that INSANE? I literally lost about half of my entire body. That's a little freaky, even.

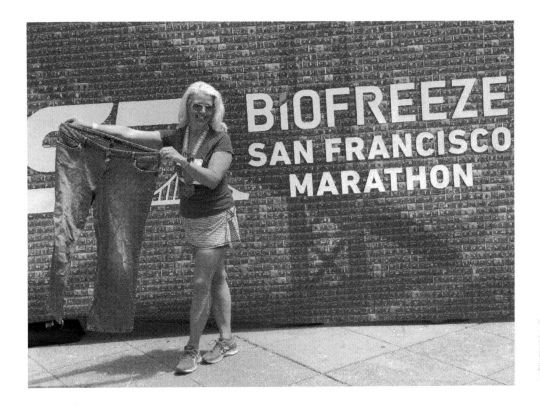

The weirdest part, I admit (I don't want to jinx myself here) was that *it wasn't that hard*. Please don't slam the book shut at this point and run screaming from the room yelling, "This girl is CRAAAAAAAZY!" I'm being serious. Once I figured out what I was doing (like how to read a nutrition label), the whole thing just flowed for me. Yes, there were obstacles along the way, but looking at the big picture here... I quickly realized that this was a way I could really eat, *like forever*, and be happy! I'm betting you can do this too with great success.

Let's get specific now. For starters, I didn't write anything down. I didn't track anything with an app or even a pencil. In hindsight I realize I might have tempted fate with that strategy! I think I might have PTSD from my Weight Watchers® days where I calculated and documented points in an official booklet. That made me crazy, I'll tell you. I would lie and cheat, borrow and steal (from myself, mind you) with that stupid tracker, and this time, I didn't want a repeat performance. That was me, though, and not you. I recommend you do whatever method will keep you, in all your honest glory, accountable. If you need to write down every morsel of what you're eating to be successful, then you should definitely do it!

Now what about the other "macros" besides counting carbs? I'll be honest here. Other than focusing on 20-50 carbs a day, I didn't count anything else, not a calorie, nor a fat gram (that's lazy keto, folks). I didn't have a "goal" or a "minimum" to achieve each day for fats or proteins. I did aim to increase my protein at every meal, and I did eat a lot of fat, which I'll go into in more detail later. For now, though, I'm trying to give you a broad picture of what I did and why I think it was successful.

Is there a reason why I didn't count fat or protein grams? Or impose goals or limits? Well for me, all that counting and tracking just sounded crazy, exhausting, and intimidating. I was already having a lifestyle adjustment by breaking up with the love of my life, carbohydrates. Piling on more rules or expectations sounded overwhelming and could be one more excuse for me to give up. Besides, what I was doing was already working -- I was losing weight!

Prior to eating DIRTY, LAZY, KETO, I probably ate 500-1000 carbs a day. I'm guessing here, but I suspect my daily intake was ridiculously high. Pasta, bread, cereal, rice... the staples in my frugal family diet were dominated by carbs. Ironically, I actually considered myself a healthy eater. I didn't eat junk food or frequent drive thrus. I only drank Diet Coke® and often snacked on baby carrots or bags of "whole wheat" Crunchy Corn Bran for cryin' out loud.

I was ignorant about how carbs affected my mood or energy level. Unbeknownst to me, every time I ate a carb-rich food, my body went into overdrive producing glucose and a quick spike in my blood sugar. In my brain, dopamine was released. The immediate physical response from eating carbs was (*and still is!*) pure, unadulterated pleasure. This positive physical reaction is why we keep eating carbs!

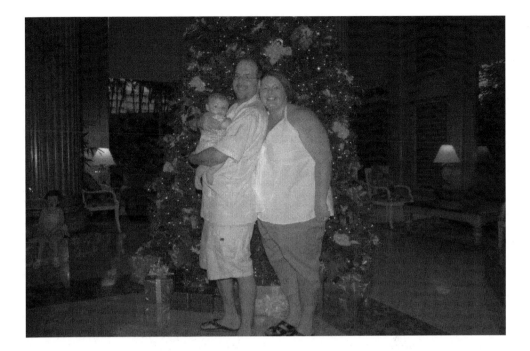

This pleasurable response, however, is short lived. Massive amounts of insulin are secreted to counteract the high blood sugar levels, leading my body to store the glucose as fat. Well, that's not fair! Then, to make matters even more complicated, the lowered blood sugar level lead to moodiness, and a desire to eat again, causing the entire cycle to repeat itself, ALL DAY LONG. No wonder I weighed so much.

Simply by reducing my carb intake within a range of 20-50 grams per day had an immediate effect on my weight and overall sense of well-being. Instead of eating a diet mainly of carbs all day, I ate lean protein and healthy fats. This new combination caused so many changes, all for the better!

Now this is what shocked the hell out of me. I suspected eating fats wouldn't be a problem (who doesn't like cheese?), but I was surprised to discover how eating more proteins at every meal was, well, *so satisfying*. I didn't find myself overeating protein like I did with simple carbs! If I ate protein at a meal or snack, I would actually feel full for longer. By choosing slow burning carbs my body surprisingly had more sustained energy. I

35

wouldn't feel sleepy after eating a meal. My frequent headaches suddenly stopped. The afternoon exhaustion, the moodiness... gone.

Whoa... Shit just got real, excuse my language.

> *The dramatic improvement in my overall health - not just with weight loss - compels me to share my story.*

If I can help even one person climb out of the carbohydrate laden hole that they have dug themselves into, out from the horrible cycle of feeling like crap all the time, then this will all have been worth it. (Sorry, starting to well up a bit here).

In addition to helping with weight loss (and afterward, maintaining your weight loss), DIRTY, LAZY, KETO will provide you with more energy than you've ever had before.

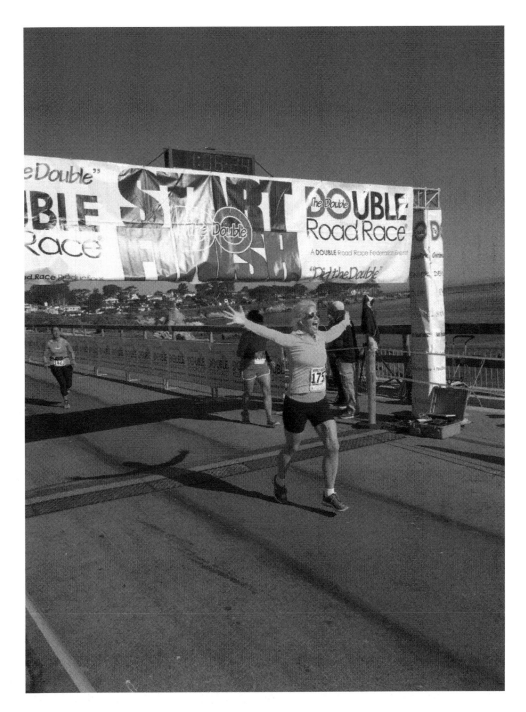

COUNTING CALORIES, COUNTING CARBS AND COMMON SENSE

> *Expect to eat between 20-50 carbs per day to lose weight, but make these carbs COUNT. Choose "slow-burning carbs" for healthy, sustainable weight loss.*

I n personal experience, when I focused on eating within a range of 20-50 grams of carbohydrates per day, I lost weight. I would like to reiterate that I did not count calories and I did not count protein or fat grams. I simply focused on the net carb count, with a sprinkling of common sense. Folks in keto-land call this version of events, "lazy keto". Further, because I allow myself to enjoy sugar-free or low carb substitutions in my regimen, I self-proclaim my eating style "dirty" (plus, it makes me feel cool). Welcome to DIRTY, LAZY, KETO!

Everyone starts differently on a DIRTY, LAZY, KETO diet. Some of us have more weight to lose than others. Because of that variability, you are likely going to have to experiment with the number of carbs you eat to see what number is going to work best for you. If you are starting at a higher weight, like I did, you might get away with eating 50 grams of carbs per day while still losing weight! Lucky you! Score one for the big girls and boys! Conversely, those with less to lose might have to eat less carbs per day to see results.

Common sense needs to play a role here. You have to be realistic about your lifestyle, activity level, and family habits. Folks that have less to lose, or are much less active, might need to focus on the lower end of the carb spend range at 20 grams per day. Either way, you don't want to go under that range of carb intake. Less is not more. I hear about dieters trying to "game the system" and eat zero carbs with a diet of beef and butter. First of all, GROSS! Now before you go defrosting some ground round, please stop and think about what you are doing. Here is the common-sense piece we talked about earlier.

> *The goal here is long term, healthy, sustainable weight loss, not some artificial, metabolic forced change that lasts only as long as you can tolerate eating BEEF AND BUTTER.*

Personally, I felt empowered eating within that range of 20-50 carbs per day. I liked the flexibility it gave me to eat out, enjoy a variety of foods, and most importantly, still feel like a "normal person" (whatever that is?).

How you "spend your carbs" is up to you, but I would like to offer you some advice from the trenches. Now I don't want to ruffle your feathers, but I have an important question for you to think about: is DIRTY, LAZY, KETO a short term or a long-term solution for your weight problem?

I'm going to assume you want to lose weight and keep it off ***for-evah***?

> *Yes, you can spend your 20-50 grams on crappy, "nutritionless" food choices that taste good in the moment (pretty much anything in a box, can, bar or pouch), but ultimately, it may catch up to you. What am I talking about here? Protein bars coated in fake chocolate, low carb ice cream, keto-friendly chips... pretty much everything you ate "before" can now be bought for a pretty penny a-la "keto-friendly" on Amazon.*

Do I ever eat these instant foods from a box, can, pouch, or bar? Why, YES, I DO! This is DIRTY, LAZY, KETO after all. But, *not all the time*. I consider these to be "**treats**" or "**emergency foods**". They don't make up my whole diet. I'm not militant about it or anything, as I eat this stuff too; however, I know that my success in losing so much weight, and in keeping it off for so long now, is that I don't eat processed foods all day long like I used to. Most of my diet now consists of real foods, like meats, cheese, eggs, vegetables, nuts, and some fruits. I don't want to scare you off or anything, but, this process took time. I just want to give you an idea of what the end-game looks like.

> *The light at the end of the tunnel is bright green, and SURPRISE, filled with vegetables!*

I know, I know, this is DIRTY, LAZY, KETO, and technically, you can eat whatever you want, but I am urging you to consider **my personal secret-sauce** for making weight loss sustainable.

Learn to eat vegetables! Ha! Were you expecting some other answer?

> *If you plan on sustaining your weight loss and turning your life around, the sooner you get over any vegetable anxiety the better.*

Vegetables are seriously the magic elixir to make your weight loss dreams come true. Romance them and get to know your vegetables. Dress them up in butter, ghee, oil, cheese, sour cream... ANYTHING to get you to eat vegetables.

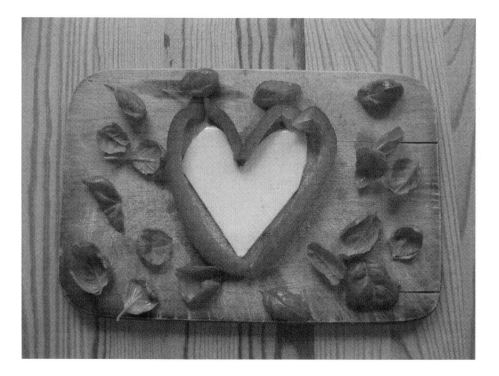

Eat vegetables as if your life depends on them. They are full of fiber and life sustaining vitamins and minerals that will prevent illness, keep you full, and melt your weight off. Vegetables are slow burning carbs and will work wonders with your metabolism.

Done. Off the soap box now.

FOOD LABELS, NET CARBS, AND SUGAR ALCOHOLS

R eading a food label under the DIRTY, LAZY, KETO rules might be different from what you've been taught. Before I send you out into the real world of eating, let's test our knowledge. In my version of keto-land, net carbs are counted by subtracting any grams of fiber and/or sugar alcohols from the listed amount of total carbohydrates. *(Why? Fiber and sugar alcohols are not digested the same as the rest of the carbohydrates as they move very quickly through your digestive system.)* Now multiply that number by the serving size that you eat. The ending quotient is your net carb. This is what you "count" in your daily allotment.

Nutrition Facts

Serving Size 3 pieces (16g)
Servings Per Container 4

Amount Per Serving

Calories 50   Calories from Fat 20

% Daily Value*

Total Fat 2.5g	4%
Saturated Fat 1g	5%
Trans Fat 0g	
Cholesterol 0mg	0%
Sodium 30mg	1%
Total Carbohydrate 9g	3%
Dietary Fiber 0g	0%
Sugars 0g	
Sugar Alcohol 8g	
Protein 1g	

Vitamin A 0% • Vitamin C 0%
Calcium 0% • Iron 0%
* Percent Daily Values are based on a 2,000 calorie diet

INGREDIENTS: Polyol...
Contains Fresh...
Tocopherol an...

I would like to remind you that "allowing" sugar alcohols is unique to the DIRTY, LAZY, KETO Diet. Many dieters that follow "true Keto" find them distasteful or downright dangerous. I would like to tip my hat in acknowledgement to all critics at this point. To address all the neigh-sayers, I would like to climb back onto my soap box for a moment.

First of all, the FDA has determined sugar alcohols and sugar substitutes are deemed GRAS (Generally Recognized As Safe). They are approved for use in this great nation of ours. I understand that this US stamp of approval doesn't mean sugar alcohols are healthy or nutritious. That being said, I am willing to take my chances. I believe that without these "sugar crutches" the alternative (FOR ME) might be obesity. Obesity comes with its own set of detrimental health issues, so I am going to pick between the two evils.

Sugar alcohols are not perfect by any means. Some cause unanticipated reactions. As long as sugar alcohols or sugar substitutes do not cause you any dietary distress (flatulence, diarrhea, etc.), then I support your common-sense approach to using them as a tool to help you lose weight. Additionally, if you find these ingredients cause an increase in your hunger/sugar cravings, then discontinue their use or limit your exposure.

I wish I could eat real sugar in safe amounts, I really do. Sadly, I cannot. I completely lose control and am not able to stop myself from overeating anything that is sweet. Even at my current healthier weight, I sometimes crave sugary treats. I am still an emotional eater, a stress eater, and even a celebratory eater, and by choosing to incorporate some sugar alcohols and sugar substitutes as they are needed (in moderation), I am able to maintain my weight loss.

DIRTY, LAZY, KETO FOOD PYRAMID

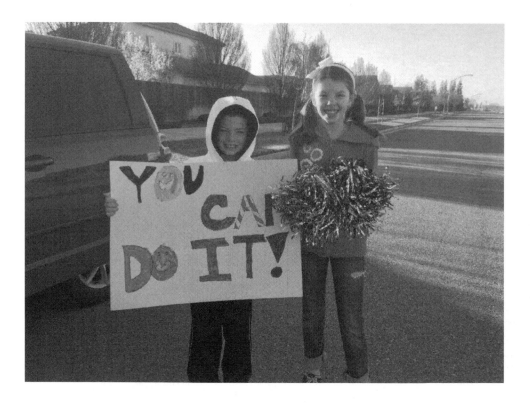

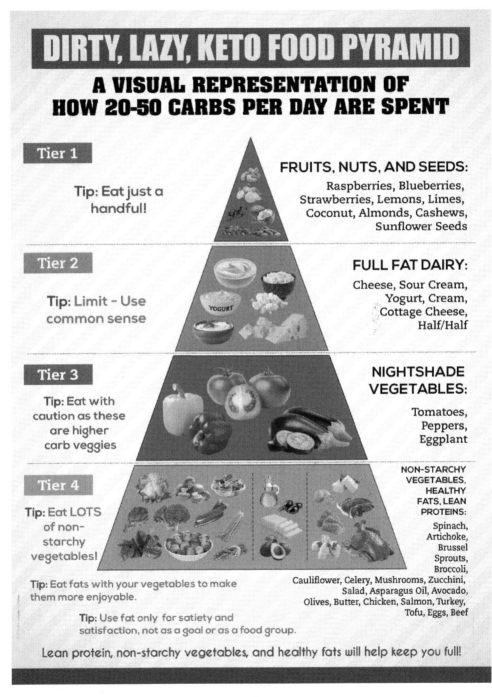

DIRTY, LAZY, KETO FOOD PYRAMID

A VISUAL REPRESENTATION OF HOW 20-50 CARBS PER DAY ARE SPENT

Tier 1

Tip: Eat just a handful!

FRUITS, NUTS, AND SEEDS:
Raspberries, Blueberries, Strawberries, Lemons, Limes, Coconut, Almonds, Cashews, Sunflower Seeds

Tier 2

Tip: Limit – Use common sense

FULL FAT DAIRY:
Cheese, Sour Cream, Yogurt, Cream, Cottage Cheese, Half/Half

Tier 3

Tip: Eat with caution as these are higher carb veggies

NIGHTSHADE VEGETABLES:
Tomatoes, Peppers, Eggplant

Tier 4

Tip: Eat LOTS of non-starchy vegetables!

NON-STARCHY VEGETABLES, HEALTHY FATS, LEAN PROTEINS:
Spinach, Artichoke, Brussel Sprouts, Broccoli, Cauliflower, Celery, Mushrooms, Zucchini, Salad, Asparagus Oil, Avocado, Olives, Butter, Chicken, Salmon, Turkey, Tofu, Eggs, Beef

Tip: Eat fats with your vegetables to make them more enjoyable.

Tip: Use fat only for satiety and satisfaction, not as a goal or as a food group.

Lean protein, non-starchy vegetables, and healthy fats will help keep you full!

DIRTY, LAZY, KETO FOOD PYRAMID

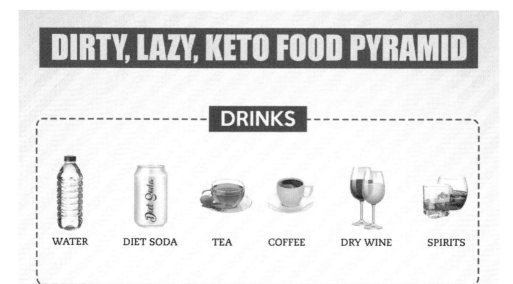

DRINKS

WATER   DIET SODA   TEA   COFFEE   DRY WINE   SPIRITS

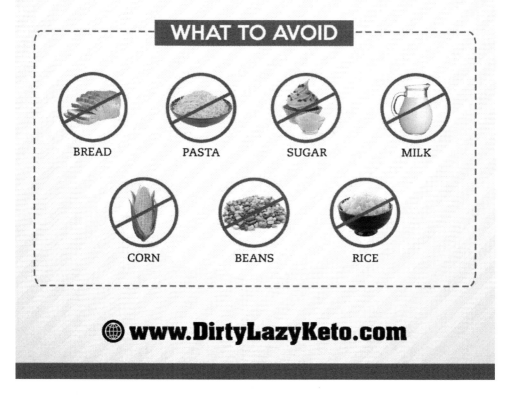

WHAT TO AVOID

BREAD   PASTA   SUGAR   MILK

CORN   BEANS   RICE

www.DirtyLazyKeto.com

FOOD PYRAMID DISCUSSION:

D o you remember blankly staring at the side of a cereal box as a child? I can clearly recall the brightly colored USDA recommendations listed adjacent to the box top offers. The tiered approach from DIRTY, LAZY, KETO, however, will likely be opposite in terms of its eating recommendations. Instead of eating the USDA's 6-8 servings of grains and cereals for example, the keto pyramid highlights the value of eating healthy fats, lean protein, and starchy vegetables.

There are a million keto pyramid guides on Pinterest, but not one DIRTY, LAZY, KETO pyramid. In fact, I made this one up! I even hired a graphic designer to make it pretty for you. If you are familiar with the "real deal" ketogenic diet, where upwards of 70% of calories stem from fat, you will immediately notice that my pyramid is different. Instead of asking you to eat fat, fat, and more fat, I am recommending you enjoy the majority of calories from healthy fat, lean protein, and non-starchy vegetables. In fact, I would like to stress that eating those three things will bring you the most success in your weight loss journey. This was how I lost 140 pounds, in a nutshell! Yes, I did enjoy full fat dairy, and some nuts, seeds, and fruit, **but the majority of my diet consists of those three big categories: healthy fat, lean protein, and non-starchy vegetables.**

An overall theme of the DIRTY, LAZY, KETO food pyramid is to eat **less net carbohydrates**. By keeping your blood sugar stable, you will stop the spikes/crashes/overeating. There is a method to the madness, people! The results of following the DIRTY, LAZY, KETO diet are stunning.

You might get angry or have a strong reaction to some of the identified food servings. It's totally normal to question the keto pyramid of eating as it's so completely different from what we were shown as children. You might even start yelling at me, "HOW CAN FRUIT MAKE ME FAT?" I understand. At first glance, this seems potentially confusing and even unfair. How have we been taught the "wrong" information for so long? Or is this just a "loophole" for losing weight? Honestly, who the hell cares? I lost half of my entire body weight following the DIRTY, LAZY, KETO diet and have kept it off for five years. I bet you can too. Let's get over ourselves and start to figure out logistics, okay?

The pyramid is supposed to give you a "visual representation" of what your overall eating in a day might look like. This is not an exact science. You do not have to "check the box" for each category. Unlike other keto programs with targeted goals/limits/ratios, with DIRTY, LAZY, KETO, the carbs are yours to spend *how you see fit*. That's what makes this program sustainable, in my opinion. That being said, I'd like to give you a broad explanation about what your eating patterns *might look like*. Do I need to say that again? This is your life. Eat what makes sense to you! With common sense and a personal mission to change your eating habits, use the keto pyramid as inspiration for your choices.

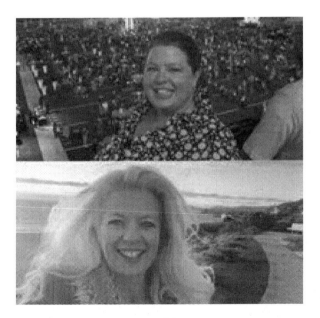

Tier 1: Just a Handful

Fruits

Starting at the top of the pyramid, you will see that keto folks eat only a few servings of fruits. This is not because fruits are bad for you; I'm not saying that at all! Fruits are delicious but naturally sweet. Because of the natural sugar, fruits are carbohydrate dense. We have discussed how high carbohydrate foods can cause blood sugar to spike/crash which often starts the cycle of eating again to improve one's energy level.

That being said, if you love eating watermelon for example, a higher carbohydrate fruit, you can still eat some freaking watermelon! This is your life and you need to make DIRTY, LAZY, KETO work for you. Don't quit a "diet" because a food isn't listed as "allowable".

> *Recognize, however, that what you "love to eat" might have a metabolic effect that causes an undesirable chain reaction.*

Even when I eat too much of something "healthy" like fruit, my energy level quickly rises when the fructose (sugar) in fruit is quickly converted by my body into glucose for immediate energy use. If I don't "burn up" that energy quickly (like with exercise), the excess glucose is stored as fat. Do I have to keep saying this throughout the mini-guide, or can you agree I'm onto something here?

My suggestion is to think of berries or low carb fruits like a "topping" not a food group. They can be enjoyed, but in small amounts. A few berries on top of yogurt, or a handful within a smoothie might provide all the natural sweetness you need to get through a craving. *The carb count per cup is for reference only, not a suggestion for you to eat an entire cup! Enjoy a sprinkle or small handful.*

Keto-Friendly Fruit Ideas[2]:

Raspberries, 7 net carbs/cup
Blueberries, 18 net carbs/cup
Strawberries, 8 net carbs/cup
Blackberries, 6 net carbs/cup
Rhubarb, 3 net carbs/cup
Starfruit, 4 net carbs/cup
Lemon, 4 net carbs/medium lemon
Lime, 5 net carbs/medium lime
Avocados (How weird is that?), 1 net carb/2.4 oz
Coconut (Also a nut and seed. Again, weird!), 5 net carbs, 1 cup shredded

---

[2] Carb counts referenced throughout this book were pulled from the 2018 Carb Manager App.

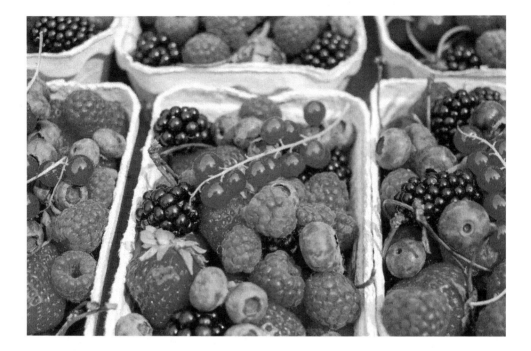

Nuts and Seeds

Also, in the "limit" range are nuts and seeds. I could eat these suckers all day long! Nuts and seeds are calorie dense and easy to over-eat (common sense!), so these land at the top of the pyramid. Even with the added fiber, it's hard to stop eating these. This is not a complete list, but something to get you started. *Note the net carbs are per cup – that doesn't mean I suggest you eat an entire cup of nuts! I'm just giving you information to consider. Enjoy just a small handful.*

Keto-Friendly Nut Ideas:

Hazel Nuts, 8 net carbs/cup
Brazil Nuts, 6 net carbs/cup
Pecans, 4 net carbs/cup
Macadamia Nuts, 6 net carbs/cup
Almonds, 14 net carbs/cup
Coconut, 5 net carbs/cup shredded (this is a fruit AND a nut)

Keto-Friendly Seed Ideas:

Chia, 12 net carbs/cup (can be constipating, beware!)
Flax, 2 net carbs/cup (can be constipating, beware!)
Pumpkin, 10 net carbs/cup
Sesame, 12 net carbs/cup
Sunflower, 19 net carbs/cup

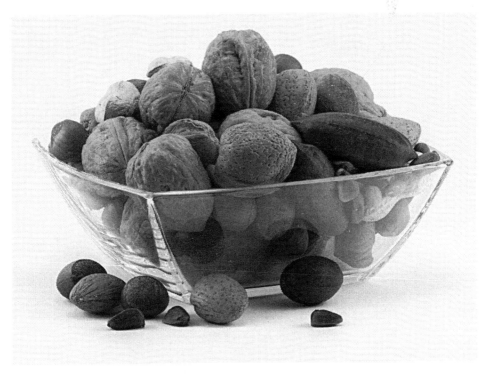

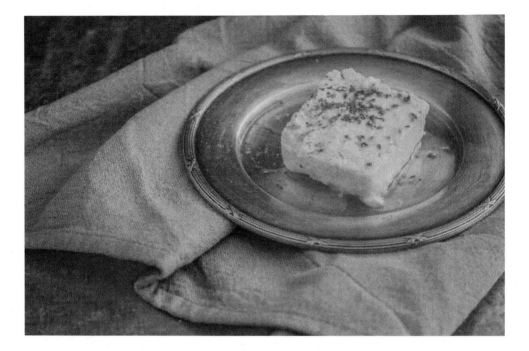

Tier 2: Full Fat Dairy

D elicious dairy! Yogurt, milk, cheese, and cream -- SERIOUSLY! How can all of this deliciousness be on a diet? So exciting, people. If you have any anger about losing your beloved pasta, please take a moment and thank the dairy category for making the hit list of DIRTY, LAZY, KETO!

Considering your daily carb spend per day is between 20-50 grams (depending on your body type, activity, and what is working best for your lifestyle), you have to be careful when consuming dairy, nuts, seeds, and fruits. Because these foods are so delicious, it is easy to get to go overboard. These foods are to be enjoyed, but in moderation. To maintain healthy digestion, you need to save room in your carb spend for fibrous vegetables.

When searching for dairy foods to enjoy, here are some tips:

Yogurt:

High fat, plain yogurt has the lowest level of carbohydrates possible. I usually buy whatever is on sale and sometimes find yogurts in the 6-8 carb/serving range. Do you have to eat yogurt? No, you don't, but you'll be passing up a great source of calcium! I frequently eat yogurt and even enjoy a sprinkle of berries on top. Note this combination might add up to 10 carbs or more – I'm wild and crazy! Another breakfast favorite of mine is to mix no sugar added cocoa powder and Splenda™ into my yogurt. This sugar-free concoction reminds me of the chocolate pudding found at a restaurant salad bar. The combinations with yogurt are endless!

Milk:

Regular milk, even full fat or low fat, remains high in carbs due the lactose component. On the other hand, the alternative milk market has broadened in recent years. Yes, this drink contains carbs, but not as many as you might expect. Almond milk, cashew milk, hemp milk, and soy milk are examples of lactose-free, unsweetened "dairy" beverages. These beauties are great to have on hand for recipes or even as a smoothie mixer. Be open minded! You might surprise yourself.

Be sure to check the label of your milk alternative for specifics, but these carb counts can help guide you:

> Almond Milk, vanilla or other flavors, unsweetened, 1 net carb/cup
> Soy Milk, Plain or Original, unsweetened, 1 net carb/cup
> Cashew Milk, unsweetened, 1 net carb/cup
> Hemp Milk, unsweetened, 0 net carbs/cup

Cream:

A little goes a long way when enjoying the rich, velvety texture of cream. I can add just a splash to my coffee or smoothie for added fat and overall decadence. Unfortunately, I hear many keto followers go completely overboard with this ingredient. They drink cup after cup of HWC - heavy whipped cream (especially in their Starbucks™ coffee) and then wonder why their weight loss has stalled. Employ some common sense, people! The dairy category hovers at the top of the keto pyramid and should be consumed in moderation.

> Heavy Whipped Cream, 0 net carbs/Tablespoon
> Half/Half, 1 net carb/.5 oz (roughly a splash)
> Sour Cream, 1 net carb/Tablespoon

Cheese

Most hard cheeses weigh in between 0 or 1 net carb/serving. Interestingly, the shredded cheeses sold in convenient pouches have more carbs than blocks of cheese. Manufacturers add potato starch and cellulose fiber to keep the shredded cheese from clumping which adds to the carb count per serving. Personally, I still buy the packaged shredded cheese because of the convenience. I have learned that the carb count varies among shredded cheese packages, so I make sure to compare packages before making a purchase. Lastly, note that cheese as a category is decadent and easy to overconsume. Even though the carb count of cheese is at the lower end, I recommend enjoying small amounts. My suggestion is to sprinkle cheese all over your vegetables and protein, rather than eating cheese as a separate snack. This strategy will help you to "slow your roll" when enjoying cheese, and also make your vegetables taste better!

> Cottage Cheese, 4% milk fat, 7 net carbs/cup
> Feta Cheese, 1 net carb/ounce
> Mozzarella Cheese, 1 net carb/ounce

Cheddar Cheese, 1 net carb/ounce
Blue Cheese, 1 net carb/ounce

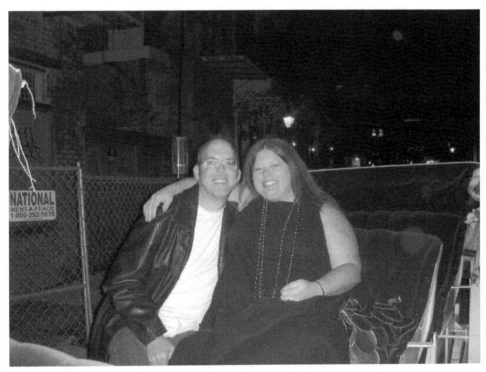

Vacations are not excuses to overeat. I try to focus on enjoying activities, not food.

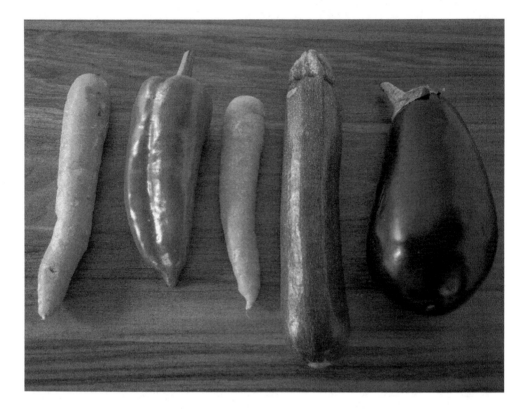

Tier 3: Are All Vegetables Good for You?

Aren't all vegetables good for you? We don't need to split hairs here, or do we? Not all vegetables are created equal. Some definitely have more carbs than others. Hello, thank you Mr. French Fry for ruining the reputation of your entire food group! Nightshade vegetables grow in the shade and flower at night. As a category, I was surprised to learn they might have more carbs than other vegetables. Examples of nightshade vegetables include eggplant, red bell peppers, tomatoes, and potatoes. Potatoes, however, offer the greatest number of carbs in the nightshade category. I do not consider potatoes to be keto-friendly. Be aware of the higher level of carbohydrates of the entire nightshade category when planning meals, recipes, and snacks. For example, I put tomatoes on my salad, but I don't eat an entire plate of tomatoes.

On a side note, some folks have negative physical reactions to eating nightshade vegetables. Reactions include diarrhea, bloating, headaches, gas, or even pain in the joints.

Keto-Friendly Nightshade Vegetables:

Tomatoes and Tomatillos, 5 net carbs/cup
Peppers
    Green Bell Peppers, 4 net carbs/cup
    Yellow Bell Peppers, 8 net carbs/cup
    Red Bell Peppers, 6 net carbs/cup
Jalapeno Peppers, 3 net carbs/cup
Eggplant, 6 net carbs/cup cooked; 2 net carbs/cup raw

Beyond the nightshade category, vegetables still vary in terms of carb count. Some argue the rule that "above ground" vegetables have less carbs than "below ground" vegetables, but even then, there are exceptions. My recommendation is to look up the nutritional value for what you are eating, and plan accordingly.

Quick tip: Did you know you can "ask Siri," "ask Google," or my favorite, "ask Alexa" for a carb count on a food? I find this more convenient than using an app.

Tier 4: Non-Starchy Vegetables

> ## *What can I binge eat?*
> ## *Non-Starchy Vegetables!*

The coffers finally start to open with the category of non-starchy vegetables. FINALLY! Eat up, sister (or brother!). Eat until your heart is content. If you're like me, you might not have a built in "off switch" when it comes to eating. I need to eat in bulk, so this is my favorite category. Find recipes that work with your lifestyle and family's needs that incorporate large amounts of non-starchy vegetables into your regime. Ideally, you want to consume these at every stinkin' meal. If it helps you swallow this information (get it, swallow!), you can coat these suckers in the fat of your choice to make them more tolerable. I hope I haven't lost you on this one. (Stay tuned, steak is coming!) I'm going to give this category a lot of air time as I can't say enough about their weight loss properties.

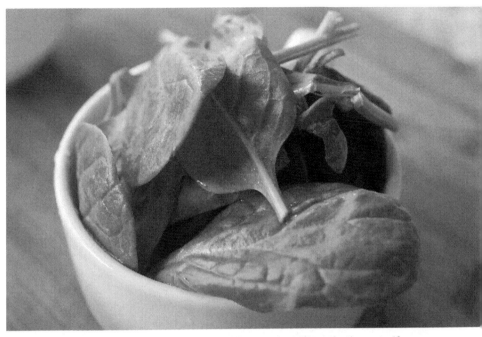

Are you a bulk eater like me? I like to fill up on greens and other cruciferous vegetables instead of chips these days. I find pairing vegetables with "dip" or "dressing" helps me stay satisfied longer.

Non-Starchy Vegetables Ideas:

Spinach, 0 net carbs/cup
Artichokes, 5 net carbs/cup
Asparagus, 2 net carbs/cup
Bamboo shoots raw, 5 net carbs/cup
Beans (Mung, green, wax, Italian), 2 net carbs/cup
Bean sprouts, 4 net carbs/cup
Brussels sprouts. 5 net carbs/cup
Broccoli, 4 net carbs/cup raw, 6 net carbs/cup cooked
Cabbage (green 3 net carbs/cup, bok choy or Chinese 1 net carb/cup)
Cauliflower, 3 net carbs/cup raw, 2 net carbs/cup cooked
Celery, 1 net carb/cup
Chayote, 4 net carbs/cup cooked
Coleslaw (greens packaged without dressing), varies per brand-estimated 3 net carbs/1.5 cups
Cucumber, 2 net carbs/cup
Daikon (Oriental Radish), 3 net carbs/cup
Greens (collard 3 net carbs/cup, kale 1 net carb/cup, mustard net carbs/cup, turnip 1 net carb/cup)
Hearts of palm, 3 net carbs/cup canned
Jicama, 5 net carbs/cup
Leeks, 7 net carbs/cup cooked, 11 net carbs/cup raw
Mushrooms, 1 net carb/cup raw
Okra, 3 net carbs/cup
Onions (white, yellow, red) 12 net carbs/cup raw, 18 net carbs/cup cooked
Pea pods (snow peas), 7 net carbs/cup
Radishes, 2 net carbs/cup
Rutabaga, 9 net carbs/cup raw, 8 net carbs/cup cooked
Salad greens (chicory 0 net carbs/cup, endive 0 net carbs/cup, escarole 0 net carbs/cup, lettuce 1 net carb/cup, romaine 1 net carb/cup, spinach 0 net carbs/cup, arugula 1 net carb/cup, radicchio 1 net carb/cup, watercress 1 net carb/cup)
Sprouts (alfalfa), 0 net carbs/cup

Zucchini, 2 net carbs/cup raw, 1 net carb/cup cooked
Sugar snap peas, 3 net carbs/cup
Swiss chard, 2 net carbs/cup cooked, 1 net carb/cup raw

Tallest bowl competition at my favorite Mongolian BBQ restaurant.

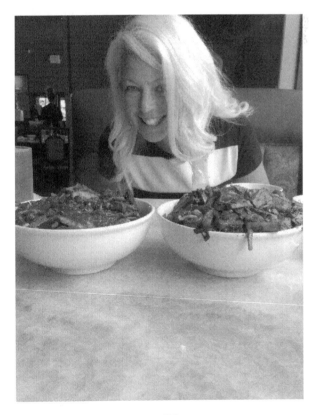

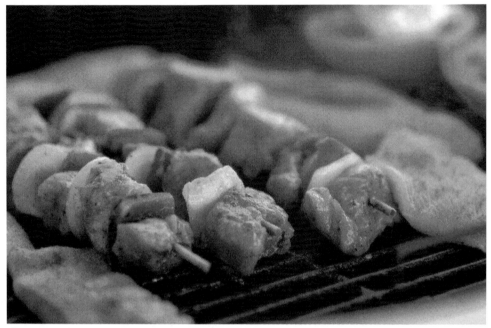

Tier 4: Protein

When I first started eating DIRTY, LAZY, KETO, something that surprised me was how little protein I was previously eating. When I changed that eating pattern and began eating protein at every meal there was an immediate positive effect. I felt more satisfied after finishing the meal, I ate less overall, and I wasn't hungry again for a while. WEIRD! My analysis is that previously I was stuck in a carbohydrate addicted cycle of false energy with no idea what sustainable energy even felt like. WOW! Let me tell you, it's a huge change for the better.

There is a wide range of proteins to meet your budget and tastes. I encourage you to eat "real food" whenever possible, and enjoy processed meat in moderation. Hot dogs and jerky, aka "keto junk food" are allowed with DIRTY, LAZY, KETO but shouldn't be the focus on your daily diet. Use common sense here to enjoy a variety of high quality proteins.

Keto-Friendly Protein Ideas:

Chicken (poultry), 0 net carbs/serving
Pork, 0 net carbs/serving
Beef, 0 net carbs/serving
Turkey, 0 net carbs/serving
Tofu, 1-2 net carbs/serving
Lamb, 0 net carbs/serving
Gyro Meat, Beef and Lamb, 5 net carbs/serving
Fish and Shellfish, 0 net carbs/serving
Duck, 0 net carbs/serving
Eggs, 1 net carbs/serving
Hot Dogs, varies per brand, estimated 2 net carbs/serving
Jerky, varies per brand, estimated 3 net carbs/serving
Lunch Meats (some have added sugar, check label)
Pepperoni, 0 net carbs/serving
Bacon, 0 net carbs/serving (check label as some have additives)
TVP Textured Vegetable Protein Meat Substitute, 1-15 net carb/serving as this varies per protein style (nuggets, crumbles, burgers, etc.)

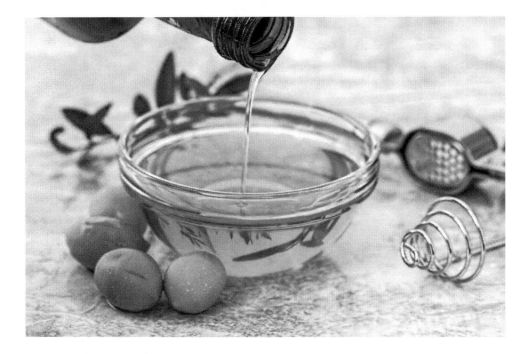

Tier 4: Healthy Fats and Oils

W ow! Who has ever told you to eat fat? I might be the first. Fat is fabulous. Fat helps everything you eat literally slide through your digestive system and out the other end! Fat is satiating and makes you feel, well, like you're not on a diet. Not feeling deprived has been critical to my success. I suspect fats are the key to why I am able to stick with DIRTY, LAZY, KETO for like five years now. I don't feel like I'm on a diet, per say. Actually, I feel pretty scandalous when I order a salad at lunch covered in blue cheese dressing, with a side of dressing! I love ordering like that, especially when I'm sitting in a restaurant with skinny "hangry" girls picking at their plain lettuce.

As a macronutrient category, I'm quite aware that there are "good fats" and "bad fats". In my own weight loss journey, I didn't discern between monosaturated fats, polyunsaturated fats and omega-3 fatty acids. I just used common sense within my families limited budget. I didn't buy Kerry Gold branded butter (considered to be the "gold standard" of keto dieters); in fact, I never even tried it. I shopped at Walmart and other discounted retailers for my groceries. I use all sorts of cooking oils, cheap mayonnaise (gasp!), generic cream cheese, half and half, and even whipping cream as my fat sources. That being said, I do encourage you to eat the healthiest fats available! This is an example of do as I say, not as I do. I aim to improve myself in this category!

Eating fat is not a goal of DIRTY, LAZY, KETO. There is no fat limit or gram counting here, just a sprinkling of common sense. You are not "required" to eat a certain amount of fat. I never did! I made sure to incorporate fats into every meal, but did not make a meal out of the fat! That is an important distinction.

> *When I hear about people eating "fat bombs" to meet a fat goal, I cringe.*

Instead, use fats to make healthy eating tolerable. Sautéing vegetables with fat, rather than eating fat for fat's sake, might offer you longer lasting results. Just sayin'.

You might be worried about how DIRTY, LAZY, KETO will affect your cholesterol levels at this point. Again, I direct you to work with your health care provider for specific guidance. I can only attest to my own personal experience when responding to this topic. Before starting DIRTY, LAZY, KETO weighing upwards of 300 pounds, my cholesterol levels were north of 300. That's not surprising, at all, right? What did floor me, however, was how dramatically my cholesterol levels dropped after losing weight while eating so much fat in the DIRTY, LAZY, KETO lifestyle. WEIRD! Since a cholesterol test is a measure of how much fat is in your blood, then why did my levels drop to "normal range"? I honestly have no idea! My doctor was also blown away. It's a Christmas miracle and I'm not about to poke holes at this magic. That's all I got on this topic, people!

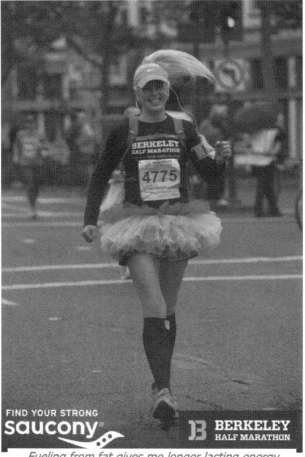

Fueling from fat gives me longer lasting energy.

Keto-Friendly Fat and Oil Ideas:

Butter, 0 net carbs/serving
Cream, 0 net carbs/serving
Ghee, 0 net carbs/serving
Oil: Coconut, Olive, etc., 0 net carbs/serving
Avocados, 1 net carbs/serving
Mayonnaise, 0 net carbs/serving
Sour Cream, 1 net carbs/serving
Cream Cheese, 2 net carbs/serving
Nuts and seeds, varies per nut or seed
Cottage Cheese, 7 net carbs/serving
Yogurt, varies per brand
Olives, 0 net carbs/serving
Coconut Milk, 8-11 net carbs/cup canned
Cheese, 0-1 net carbs/serving
Salad Dressing, depends on brand
MCT[3] Oil, 0 net carbs/serving

---

[3] *I do not use MCT oil, but if I don't mention it, I'm sure to get complaints.*

What's in Your Kitchen? Conduct the "Keto Cleanse"

N ew folks to keto often ask for advice on how to get started. Here is my number one tip. TAKE A CLOSE LOOK AT WHAT IS IN YOUR KITCHEN. If your cabinets are stocked with carbolicious snacks, you will be fighting an uphill battle. I realize your family might not be on board with DIRTY, LAZY, KETO, but then again, do they want to see you die an early death from a diabetes related complication? Didn't think so. Your family can mourn the loss of their beloved Chips-A-Hoy Cookies™ and embrace a healthier future together. Sorry for being sassy here, but this is a serious matter. If you are going to be successful on this diet, you need to remove temptations and stock your fridge and pantry shelves with easy to reach keto-friendly ingredients.

75

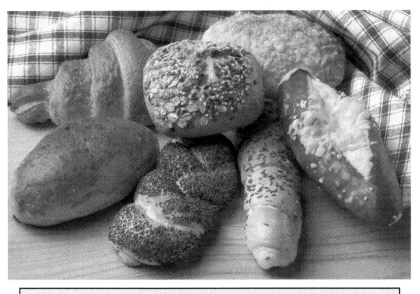

I remember searching the cabinets for "something sweet" and coming up empty. In my desperation, I gnawed on a baking square of chocolate which tasted only one notch above eating dirt.

Set yourself up for success by conducting a "Keto Cleanse" by:

*Removing high carb foods from your fridge and pantry – if it's not there, you can't eat it!
*Stop buying high carb foods at the store
*Moving high carb items to a different shelf in your pantry or fridge –making them "harder to reach" or "out of sight"

"Keto Cleanse" - Remove Tempting Foods:

Candy
Sugar
Soda (not diet)
White Flour
Mixes for brownies/cake
Pasta
Bread
Potatoes
Frozen dinners
Granola Bars
Crackers
Chips
Instant noodles
Desserts
Rice
Cereal
Canned fruit
Syrup
Corn
Muffins
Pretzels
Baked Goods
Oatmeal
Beans
Tortillas
Frozen Pizza
French Fries
Milk
Fruit Juice
Honey

Sauces or Salad dressings with more than 2 carbs per serving
Sweet Wines
Flavored Alcohols (ex. Bailey's)
Sugary Mixers for Cocktails
Chocolate (I tried to sneak this one in last so maybe you wouldn't catch it)

LET'S GO SHOPPING!

D epending on who you ask, the shopping list for a DIRTY, LAZY, KETO lifestyle is going to vary tremendously. Everyone has a different amount of time and money to devote towards grocery shopping.

> *Without making any excuses, shopping for keto-friendly foods must be a priority.*

Spending more money won't help you lose weight faster. There are no "fancy ingredients" required to make this diet work. While some folks will shop at their local farmer's market, others (like me) will go to AT LEAST five discount grocery stores to stock up on sale items and loss leaders.

> *Bottom line, no matter what your budget is, this is possible. Do not give up on losing weight because you think you can't afford it.*

Grocery Store Shopping Tips:

When you go to the grocery store, shop along the perimeter and avoid going down any aisles. (The healthy stuff is usually around the edges of the store.)

> *Do the shopping yourself. You will always get what you need and will have no one but yourself to blame.*

Buy keto-friendly ingredients slowly. Like a good wardrobe, purchase the ingredients as you need them, or as a "treat", but not all at once. For example, I buy almond flour (which I consider pricey) only once a year during the holidays. I use this to make the crust for a sugar-free cheesecake to serve at Christmas dinner.

Plan for leftovers. I find that by making a big crock pot of shredded chicken, for example, I am able to make multiple meals.

Take short cuts. This can be overwhelming! Make your life easier by including easy short cuts like buying a rotisserie chicken or premade salmon kabobs.

Don't worry about throwing vegetables away. Buy more than you think you need. VEGETABLES ARE A GREAT INVESTMENT IN YOUR HEALTH.

Bring a list.

Of course, you want to customize your shopping list depending on your budget, family needs, and overall tastes. Here are some overall concepts for you to consider as you plan what you need to get started on DIRTY, LAZY, KETO.

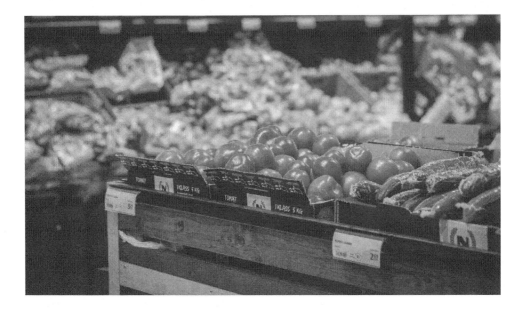

Overall Concepts for Grocery Shopping

FATS – What is your preference? Butter, Oil, Avocados, MCT oil? There you go.

PROTEIN – Lots of meat and eggs (and/or if you like, plant-based proteins)

HEALTHY SLOW BURNING CARBS – Green vegetables people!

DAIRY – Full fat yogurt, sour cream, cream, cheese, butter

NUTS & SEEDS – Just a pack or two to get you started

BERRIES – again, just a pack or two to get you started

Stephanie's Secret Shopping List

Take a picture of the list using your phone, and you will always have it with you at the store! You can enlarge the list easily by zooming in.

DIRTY, LAZY, KETO

STEPHANIE'S SECRET SHOPPING LIST

*These are not required! I'm just sharing my family grocery list with you.
I don't necessarily buy every single item on this list as I do stock up when things are on sale. This is a "working list."*

WWW.DIRTYLAZYKETO.COM

DAIRY

Unsalted Butter
Cream Cheese (full fat)
Cottage Cheese 4% milk fat
Eggs
Cheese (all kinds including parmesan)
Heavy Whipped Cream
Half and Half (full fat)
Sour Cream (full fat)
Yogurt (Plain, full-fat unsweetened - check label)
Unsweetened almond milk or other dairy alternative milk
Can of Whipped Cream (the real deal! For emergencies!)

MEATS

Chicken (Rotisserie and raw – all parts)
Seafood (whatever is on sale)
Tofu
Deli Meats (check labels as some brands add sugar)
Meats for dinner (ground turkey, sausage, steak, etc.)
Bacon
Pepperoni

PRODUCE

Avocados
Celery
Artichokes
Broccoli
Cauliflower – whole
Cauliflower – riced (in bag)
Nuts
Shredded coleslaw/cabbage mix
Berries
Lettuce and Salad Mixes
Spinach
Zucchini
Asparagus
Brussel Sprouts
Cucumbers
Onions
Lemons and Limes
Soybeans
Mushrooms
Jalapenos
Fresh herbs
Pesto

DRINKS

Diet Soda
Flavored seltzer waters
Electrolyte water (sugar free)
Non-Fat hot cocoa (strangely, this has less carbs than sugar free hot cocoa)
Low-Carb beers (examples: Michelob Ultra®, Corona Premier®)
Hard Alcohol (zero carbs)
Sugar-Free energy drinks
Tea and coffee
Sugar-Free water flavor packets (or squirts) in every flavor under the sun

BAKING

Coconut Oil, Olive Oil, Peanut Oil
Flax
Chia seeds
Protein powder
Almond flour for baking (used very rarely)
CarbQuik® Baking Powder (used very rarely)
Soy flour and coconut flour (used very rarely)
Splenda® or sugar substitute (Swerve®, Monkfruit, etc.)
Cocoa powder unsweetened

RANDOM

Olives
Peanut Butter
Sugar-Free Candy (for emergencies!)
Mayo (full fat)
Low-Carb tortillas (occasional splurge)
Sugar-Free JELLO® gelatin powders
Salad dressing (ranch, blue cheese, check label)
Pickles
Spaghetti Sauce – no sugar added
Ketchup – Sugar Free
Mustard
Hot Sauce (check label)
Bouillon cubes
Sugar-Free pancake syrup
Protein bars (occasionally, check label)
Tuna

81

Typical Meals on DIRTY, LAZY, KETO

W hat does a typical meal look like on DIRTY, LAZY, KETO? The beauty of this lifestyle is the variety. It's hard to pin-point what everyone's meals should look like as there is no "right" or "wrong" meal providing that its low carb. I can share, however, popular meals many people eat (including me) to get you started.

BREAKFAST

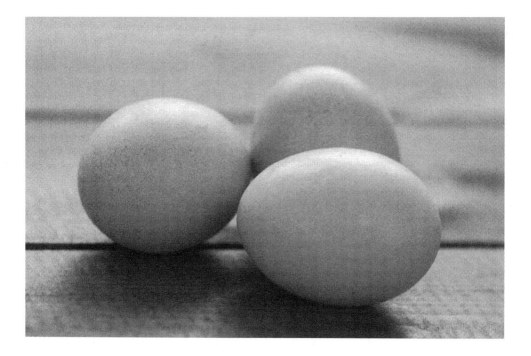

What to eat? Eggs? Bacon? Why not. Isn't this the best diet in the world? Who the hell eats bacon and loses weight? Can I get an amen, sisters and brothers? I also recommend getting in vegetables here by adding them to your omelet or egg muffins. Why am I suggesting eating vegetables in the morning? Am I crazy or something? In addition to the health component of providing vitamins and minerals (boring), the fiber in vegetables will help you stay fuller longer, and help you eat less during the actual meal.

> *I think of vegetables as a necessary "filler" to slow my eating down.*

If a hot breakfast isn't your style, maybe you would prefer cold yogurt or cottage cheese? As long as you're not reaching for toast, cereal, or oats, you can be creative in your new morning routine. Who says you can't enjoy lunch meat for breakfast? Or how about avocados?

What can you drink in the morning? I would love for you to start drinking water, water, water, water, water... but of course you'll need some coffee first! YES, COFFEE IS OKAY!

One of the most common questions I hear from new Keto diet followers is,

> *"What is bulletproof coffee and do I have to drink that?"*

The simple answer is no, you don't have to drink anything weird. **Bulletproof Coffee (BPC)** is a fancy term for coffee with some fat in it.

You will still lose weight on the keto diet *without* bulletproof coffee! But for the sake of argument, let's take a look at what it is and why so many people swear by it.

Fat, as we know, is satiating and curbs hunger. Further, some espouse that "bulletproof coffee" provides mental clarity and even starts their day with a clean boost.

Simply by changing your morning coffee from black to adding fat will help prolong eating of the first meal of the day. Many try to "fast" as long as possible between their last meal at night, and their first meal in the morning to assist with weight loss. Fat added to your morning coffee will curb your appetite, allowing you to "break the fast" with breakfast a bit later in the day.

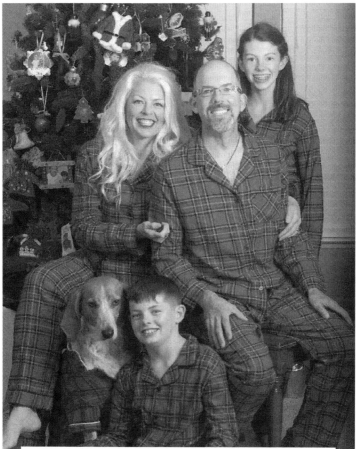

My Christmas tradition is to bake a "soufflé" while we open presents. I mix a dozen eggs with various vegetables, cheese, and bacon all in one glass dish. Once it cools, it's easy to cut into squares. Everyone is happy! Easy to make the night before too.

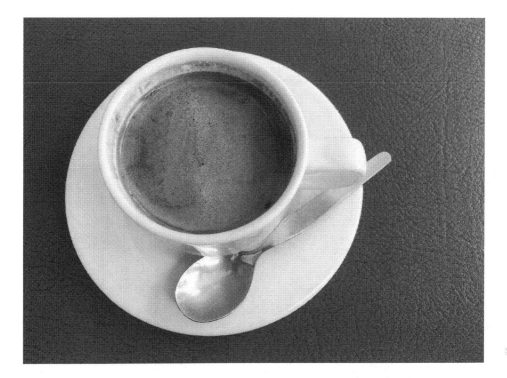

Popular Keto-friendly Coffee Additives (1-2 Tablespoons):

Unsalted Butter: Kerrygold® brand is popular, but let's be honest here, any unsalted butter will do unless you have an incredible palate. Kerrygold® branded butter is made from the cream of grass-fed Irish cows, so apparently that must taste better! Whether due to its high-quality cream or perhaps due to the current keto coffee craze, Kerrygold® brand butter is currently the third best-selling butter in the U.S.! It's sold at Wal-Mart®, Costco® and major retailers.

Ghee: clarified butter, popular with Indian cooking

Heavy Cream: (or whipping cream – NOT whipped cream, sad!) This happens to be my current personal favorite. I use half/half or whipping cream.

MCT Oil: (Commercial source would be Coconut Oil or Palm Kernal Oil): (Ohhhhhhh, controversial!) MCT oil stands for Medium Chain Triglyceride This tasteless and odorless oil has been used historically as a fat source in infant formulas, and more recently by athletes and those looking for alternative energy sources. MCT oil is easily metabolized, bypassing the intestines for digestion, heading straight to the liver. Some argue that MCT oil provides increased energy and aids in leading the body toward ketosis, the fat burning state keto dieters strive for. Side effects of digesting MCT oil might include light headedness, increased heart rate, and diarrhea, so use with caution.

What about sweeteners? Can the keto-friendly diet include a sweetened version of bulletproof coffee? The answer depends on how strictly you follow the keto diet. Diehard ketogenic followers argue against artificial sugars of any kind – they claim artificial sweeteners can wreak havoc on your blood sugar, which could derail your weight loss success. Some might focus simply on the potential health risks of consuming chemicals. Others see artificial sweeteners as a personal choice, and not a "rule" of the keto diet; there might even be value to using them as a temporary crutch to help avoid consuming sugar.

Even among artificial sweetener users there continues to be division. Many have strong opinions about which artificial sweetener is the best tasting, most natural, or safest to use. Ultimately, not everyone responds the same to artificial sweeteners, and many are able to indulge without immediate consequence.

Personally, while losing 140 pounds, I had a hard time changing my coffee routine. I was used to real-deal milk and sugar, and unwilling to let go of that sweet flavor. For years, I relied on sugar-free coffee creamers for my morning kick-start. Nestle Coffee-Mate® Sugar-Free Vanilla, Hazelnut, and Italian Sweet Cream were my favorites. When those weren't available, I would use half/half with a splash of Torani® flavored sugar-free syrup. (Note: many Sugar-Free syrups are available at Starbucks™ or even McDonalds™!) This is your body, and you get to decide whether or not to supplement your coffee. Artificial flavors, coloring, or sweeteners are allowed. DIRTY, LAZY, KETO has your back if someone wants to call in the keto police for a throw down.

It's almost comical how strongly we feel about our morning coffee. Ask any keto dieter their opinion on the matter and you most certainly will get an earful! The bottom line is that bulletproof coffee is a personal choice. Fat added to coffee is a means to help control your blood sugar. Think of bulletproof coffee as an option, not a requirement, in your DIRTY, LAZY, KETO diet.

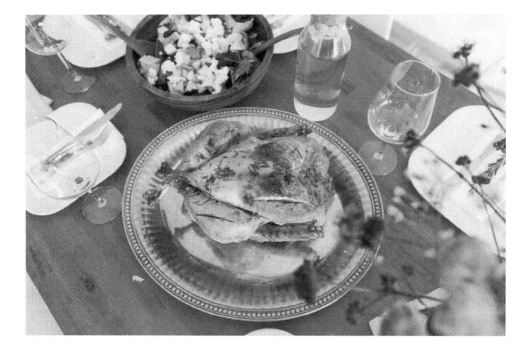

LUNCH & DINNER

I'm going to speak very generally here, but most of your DIRTY, LAZY, KETO meals will consist of some protein, some fats, and lots of non-starchy vegetables. You can mix and match combinations of the three with endless possibilities. Pinterest and Facebook will provide you with millions of free meal ideas that meet all of your parameters. On a budget? Kid- friendly? Vegan? A quick search for low carb recipes with whatever ingredients you happen to have on hand is just a few mouse clicks click away. This is not meant to be a cookbook (I'm quite lazy, remember), so I will direct you elsewhere for your gourmet recipes.

Tips for Making Meals Easy:

In the beginning, you might find it helpful to stick to a few dinners that "work for you". Just get your party started, have some success on the scale, and then branch out to add more meals. It's okay to repeat meals and add in more variety later as you learn new ideas.

It's tempting when first starting a DIRTY, LAZY, KETO diet to think that you "must have" expensive retail substitution items. Here is an example -- everyone loves pizza, right? Some snazzy marketing guy figured out there must be a demand for low carb pizza crust. He reconfigured a recipe that substituted cauliflower for white flour and is now making a boatload of money selling these crust alternatives at Target, Costco, and other major retailers. Do you have to buy these, and other "substitution items"? NO, YOU DO NOT.

I consider these a luxury item. I never used these high-priced alternatives, and I still lost weight. Can you buy them if your budget allows you to? YES, YOU CAN! In my opinion, they aren't necessary, but can be "helpful" if used appropriately. Let me explain.

There are a lot of changes in front of you. It's hard to let go of old habits, I understand! My family ate pizza every Friday night for like, one hundred years, so when I realized I had to say goodbye to that tradition, I felt left out and a bit resentful. Buying one of these pizza substitution crusts might have helped me temporarily, but in the end, I needed to develop a new routine for my Friday night that was sustainable. I didn't need to eat pizza to take part in the Friday night tradition. Spending time with my loved ones was really what mattered, not the food. Do you see where I'm going with this?

> *I found chicken wings with a salad an easy substitution for "Friday Night" pizza. Oh, and focusing on my family, rather than the food routine!*

I would like to reiterate how the retail substitution items are a "crutch" to help transition your eating from the "old" to the "new" behaviors. They are certainly "allowed" on a DIRTY, LAZY, KETO diet, but I urge you to start thinking of new ways to meet your needs at that moment that don't require an expensive specialty item that might ultimately let you down with taste, availability, or price.

DESSERTS

While desserts are definitely not a meal, many of us with a history of being overweight have treated desserts like an entree. You are not alone with your sweet tooth, my friend! The physical cravings for sugar will deter over time on the DIRTY, LAZY, KETO diet, but until we change our emotional triggers that scream "SUGAR... NOW!" there will always be a need for something sweet.

> *There is no judgement here. I come from a generation of eating Fruit-Loops™ and drinking Kool-Aid™, so clearly my blood runs thick with artificial colors and flavoring.*

Using artificial sweeteners (or natural sugar substitutions) in your diet is a personal choice. There are many to choose from, and I'm sure some are healthier than others. I'm not here to advocate which one you choose (if any), but I am going to climb on my soapbox and scream to all the members of keto-land, "GO AHEAD AND ENJOY YOUR KETO-FRIENDLY DESSERTS!".

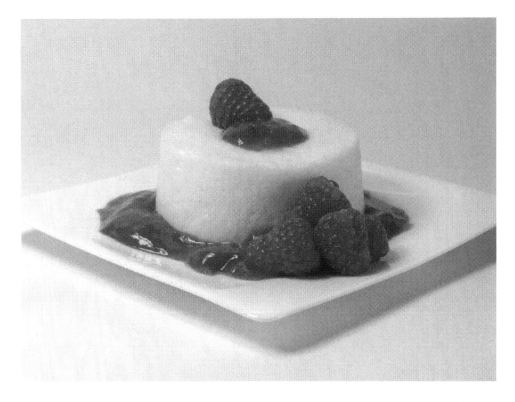

Some people get all riled up about this topic. They have VERY STRONG FEELINGS and will begin SHOUTING about their sugar belief systems. I am so curious about this. Why do folks care if I put Splenda™ on my coleslaw? I mean, really! I agree with the overall concept that sprinkling chemicals (or natural monk fruit, *whatever*) on my food might not be the best idea, but if I need that crutch to be successful at losing weight and improving my overall health in the big picture, then why isn't that okay?

There are a few things happening here that I would like to point out. First of all, I would like to question the motives of the "keto police". If a critic honestly has my best interest in mind, then stop me now and let me thank you. Not everyone is trying to be supportive, however. Some people like to criticize others simply to feel better about themselves. They are trying to prop themselves up onto a righteous high horse to create false feelings of superiority. I suspect they are sad underneath their smugness, and I believe they are struggling just like the rest of us. There is no shame in wanting something sweet. We are not weak for desiring pleasure!

Before we continue, can I stop and state the obvious here?

> *"I KNOW THIS FAKE SUGAR CRAP ISN'T GOOD FOR ME, BUT RIGHT NOW I NEED IT TO PREVENT ME FROM GIVING UP."*

All that being said, I will leave you with one final thought about sugar substitutions, natural or artificial. Even if they are low carb or altogether sugar-free, some products can trigger your blood sugar to rise and activate the sugar-craving cycle. This is so not fair! Everyone reacts differently, though, and only you can determine if sweeteners are helpful or hurtful to your success. If you find that after eating something with one of these substitutions causes you to fall back into "old patterns", then perhaps you may want to avoid that item in the future, or limit the quantity. I want you to be successful, so these are tips and advice that I have learned from my own experience.

Sugar Substitutes:

Acesulfame K (Ace-K) – Sweet One®
Advantame
Aspartame – Equal®, Nutra Sweet®, Sugar Twin®
Monk Fruit or Swingle fruit (Luo Han Guo) – Monk Fruit in the Raw®, Nectresse®, PureFruit®, PureLo®
Neotame
Saccharin – Necta Sweet®, Sweet'N Low®, Sweet Twin®
Steviol glycosides – Sweet Leaf®, PureVia Stevia®, In the Raw®, Truvia®
Sucralose – Splenda®
Organic Raw Coconut Sugar (Fresh Thyme®)

What About Flour?

For some reason, flour substitutes don't generate as much drama, despite their ability to negatively affect one's blood sugar. Perhaps this is because we don't usually "crave" flour, like we "crave" sugar? Or maybe it is because flour substitutes aren't riddled with chemicals like sugar substitutes often are. Whatever the reason, people seem more open-minded to swap out traditional white flour for something with lower carbs. All of these vary in terms of carbs per serving, taste, and performance within a recipe, so do your research before replacing white flour in your food preparation.

Examples of Flour Substitutes:

Almond Flour, 2 net carbs/.5 cup
Coconut Flour, 3-12 net carbs/.5 cup, depending on brand
Soy Flour, 6-9 net carbs/.5 cup, depending on brand
Flax Meal, 0-2 net carbs/Tablespoon, depending on brand
Phyllium Husk, 0-1 net carbs/Tablespoon, depending on brand
Low Carb Baking Mix, varies per brand

SNACKS

I exist in a constant state of anxiety and fear that I will find myself in an unexpected location without keto-friendly food. It's true that I also have irrational thoughts of a single hunger pang leading to uncontrollable carbohydrate "binge-eating".

> *I definitely don't want my lack of planning to be a reason for me to "fall off the wagon" and end up snacking on a dozen churros!*

Because of my deep-seeded fears, you will always find my purse stuffed with secret DIRTY, LAZY, KETO snacks.

> *To this day, my coworkers tease me about a time we were traveling for work, and the T.S.A. inspector identified and inspected "suspicious items" in my carry-on luggage, a Ziplock® of turkey bacon and an avocado!*

Whether I'm driving across country, sitting through a long meeting, or taking a walk around the block, I've been known to have an excessive amount of options to enjoy. Plan for success, people.

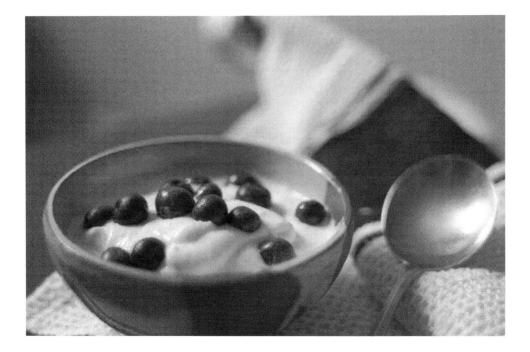

Keto-Friendly Snack Ideas:

Hard-boiled eggs
Celery
Yogurt
Beef Jerky
Bacon
Raw, sliced vegetables
String Cheese
Pickles
Olives
Pork Rinds
Avocado Slices
Deli Meat
Cubed Cheese
Seaweed Snacks
Fried Cubed Tofu
Nuts
Sugar-Free Jell-O™ cups
Protein Bar
Water, water, water, water

DRINKS

In addition to drinking your water, water, water, water, DIRTY, LAZY, KETO supports your decision to drink diet soda. GASP! You can even enjoy alcohol that is low carb or zero carb. WOW! AGAIN, BEST DIET EVER! Black coffee and tea are zero carb too. Because your carbs are yours to spend, you can even choose almond milk or dairy alternative milks to enjoy that are low enough in carbohydrates to slip into your smoothies. Because I like to focus on what you CAN HAVE and not want you CAN'T, I'm *not* going to focus on the long list of sugary beverages that have more carbs in one cup than you will eat in an entire day. Those drinks are a thing of the past. Let's talk about our current options.

ZERO CARB Drink Ideas:

Water
Seltzer Water (sugar free)
Electrolyte Water (Mio™, Powerade™, Smart Water™)
Mineral Water or naturally flavored water
Black Coffee (or with full fat cream)
Tea (herbal, black, green)
Diet-Soda
Sugar-free Energy Drinks (check label as some still contain carbs)
Soda water (NOT TONIC)
Hard Alcohols[4]: Whiskey, Scotch, Rum, Brandy, Cognac, Vodka, Tequila, Gin

---

[4] *I hesitate to provide carb information about servings of alcohol as who consumes only one serving? Because there are no nutrition labels on alcohol, I wanted to provide carb information here. This information may not be 100% accurate as brands and styles of alcohol vary greatly. Be forewarned, however, as the more alcohol one drinks, the less likely you are to give a crap about following DIRTY, LAZY, KETO!*

LOW CARB Drink Ideas:

Lemon or Lime added to water (carb counts depend on how much you add)

Low Carb Energy Drinks

Dairy Alternative Drinks (ex. Unsweetened Almond Milk, Coconut Milk, Cashew Milk, Flax Milk, Hemp Milk, Soy Milk – check the label for carb count)

Bone Broth

Vegetable Smoothies

Protein Smoothies

Coffee with additives that contain carbs (like Sugar-Free Creamers)

Champagne (1.5 carbs)

Red Wine: Pino Noir (3.4 carbs), Merlot (3.7 carbs), Cabernet Sauvignon (3.8 carbs)

White Wine*: Sauvignon Blanc (3 carbs), Pinot Grigio (3 carbs), Chardonnay (3.2 carbs)

Light Beer: Bud Select® 55 (1.8 carbs), Bud Select® (3.1 carbs), Michelob Ultra® (2.6 carbs), Michelob Ultra Amber® (3.2 carbs), Amstel Light® (5 carbs)

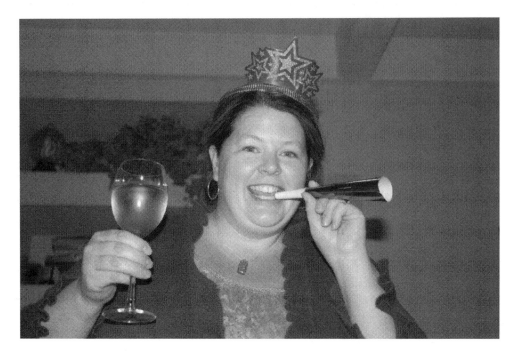

Beware of the carbs in your drink!

Myths about DIRTY, LAZY, KETO

KETO FLU

Nothing would make me sadder than to hear that you quit DIRTY, LAZY, KETO because you weren't prepared for the changes ahead. I would like to address common myths about starting a ketogenic diet, and specifically, help you prevent the mythical "keto flu" from coming on.

When you change your body's main fuel source from carbohydrates to fats/proteins, you must expect a transition period. If you were like me, and enjoyed hundreds upon hundreds of carbs per day, your body was used to sugar being pumped through the veins almost nonstop. This is a carbohydrate addicted cycle of false energy! When you stop mainlining

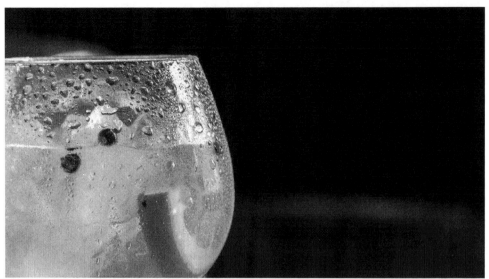

sugar and carbohydrates you might suddenly feel a change in your energy patterns. I believe this is normal! Give your body a chance to breathe and learn to trust its new fuel source. You might even want to "give yourself a break" from work-outs as your body adjusts. Everyone reacts differently, but most people bounce back within a week or two.

> *The mythical "keto flu" is the number one reason people quit the keto diet.*

There will be times in the day you might just feel tired. That is okay! Maybe your body is saying, "hey, I need a break right now." I definitely experienced this. I was used to eating carbs whenever I felt tired, so I had to learn how to stop fighting those feelings and just let my body feel tired. Feeling tired sometimes is a normal part of the day and doesn't need to be "fixed" with stimulants like sugary coffee or carbs for immediate energy. Consider getting more sleep at night, taking an afternoon siesta, or scheduling a mediation break in lieu of high carb snacking to refresh your energy levels.

In addition to experiencing changes in your energy levels, when you are losing weight, you are also changing your body's composition of water weight. While I never personally experienced any adverse health symptoms related to dehydration, I want to forewarn you of the possible consequences if you don't take this section seriously. Dehydration is a serious medical condition which requires medical intervention. You must anticipate your body's increased need for water by dramatically increasing your daily intake of fluids.

Symptoms of Metabolic Electrolyte Deficiency Syndrome:

*Heart palpitations or racing heart
*Fatigue
*Dizziness or shakiness
*Headaches or migraines
*Leg cramps or other muscles cramps, especially at night
*Constipation or a feeling of uncomfortable bloating
*Nausea or vomiting

To avoid dehydration symptoms, your body requires additional water and electrolytes. Electrolytes will prevent you from feeling tired and experiencing the mythical "keto flu." Without getting all "scientific" (yup, that word again), I want to give you a quick run-down. Electrolytes are minerals such as sodium, potassium, calcium and magnesium; they balance the amount of water in your body to help your cells function properly by removing waste products. Do you need to know any of the specifics? Nope. You do, however, need to take personal responsibility to increase the number of electrolytes in your diet.

Boost Electrolytes in Your Diet by Consuming:

*Bone broth

*Consuming sports drinks that include electrolytes (example, Sugar-Free Powerade®)

*Adding NUUN® sugar-free tablets to your water (full disclosure, I currently volunteer as an Ambassador for the brand NUUN® without any commission or compensation)

*Eat foods rich in potassium (nuts, salmon, avocados, leafy green veggies and mushrooms)

*Eat foods rich in calcium (dairy foods like yogurt or cheese, leafy green vegetables, broccoli, fish, almond or coconut milk, canned salmon, shrimp, and peanuts)

*Drink water, water, water, water

*Supplementation of electrolytes via tablets (under advisement of your doctor)

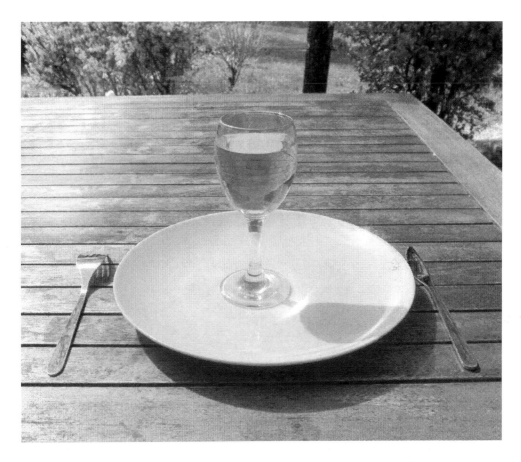

Is Intermittent Fasting Required?

I ntermittent Fasting is getting a lot of air time lately in the media. Doctors love to glom onto a new idea that could "save the world" from obesity. They claim that fasting, or greatly reducing caloric intake for an extended period of time can improve metabolism, decrease insulin resistance, and help you lose stubborn belly fat. Who am I to argue with such a miraculous discovery?

Of course, I have a lot to say about this matter. Telling an overweight person to just "stop eating" sounds a lot like the shaming calorie-restrictive diets that I grew up with. While I'm sure that the science behind this technique is entirely accurate, I predict problems with its implementation.

Fasting means we can't eat for a period of time. But when we are told we can't do something, the rebel inside of us immediately wants to break that rule. **This is where I see a problem.**

> *When dieters "break a rule," they feel guilty. Guilty feelings are wrapped in shame, and shameful feelings manifest as negative self-talk, leading to self-sabotage.*

Examples of Self-Sabotage:

*I can't do this.
*This is too hard.
*I'm not strong enough.
*I don't have will power.
*Forget it. I just caved in.

Before you know it, the fasting dieter has lost all of their confidence and decides they aren't capable of sticking with the program. Because of this negative, shameful experience, they revert back to old behaviors of comfort eating for solace.

DIRTY, LAZY, KETO wants you to be successful. You don't need to fast or deprive yourself to lose weight. Sure, this research might sound promising, but if you aren't able or willing to conduct "intermittent fasts", you can still lose weight!

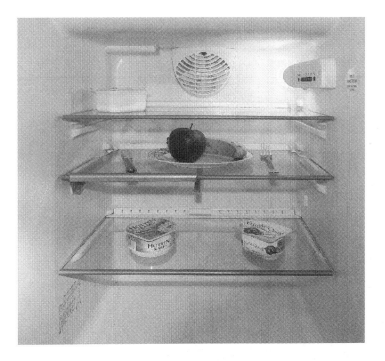

You might wonder if I incorporated fasting into my own personal weight loss experience? Unintentionally, I discovered there are benefits of taking breaks with my eating. I found that the evening "mini-fast" works best for me. I stop eating at dinner-time and resume my Olympic level eating the next day at breakfast.

> *Making a cold "stop" of eating after dinner has helped me avoid those dark hours of nonstop binge-eating in front of the television.*

When I made this "rule" for myself about not eating in the evenings, it wasn't motivated by current research about resetting my metabolism. I was trying to stop unwanted behavior. You will have to see what works best for you!

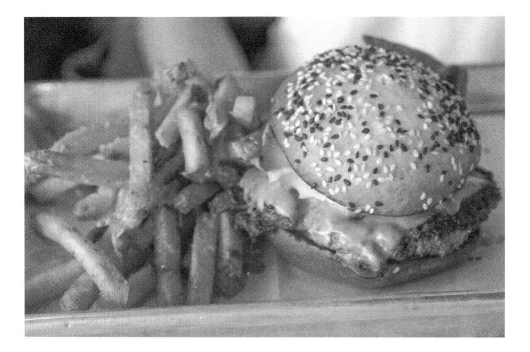

Cheat Days or Cheat Meals

Are you serious about sustainable, long-term weight loss? Or is this only a temporary ploy only for showing off your figure at an upcoming social event? I'm hoping you are committed about making permanent changes toward living a better life. Cheat meals or cheat days will wreak havoc on your weight loss. They will confuse your metabolism and derail your confidence. There is a physical and emotional momentum to your weight loss, and I urge you to reconsider any plans to backtrack.

There are so many excuses that, on the surface, sound totally legitimate. I urge you to recognize the idiocity of your "old self" trying to sabotage your progress. Here are some examples of the lies we tell ourselves. Feel free to pencil in your own thoughts here, as I know we all become extremely creative when lying to ourselves!

Common Excuses for Cheating

I deserve this.
YOLO – You only live once.
Holidays don't count.
It's my birthday (or another holiday).
This isn't fair. I want to eat like everyone else.
Vacations are an exception.
I don't want to hurt the feelings of my hostess.
I've had a bad day.
I'll go to the gym after
My body is just built this way.
This is too expensive.
I deserve a treat.
I shouldn't be eliminating food groups – it's not natural.
I'm fine just the way I am. I don't need to lose weight.
I need a break once and a while.
My husband/wife/partner isn't supporting me.
I'll start tomorrow.
This food is part of my family's tradition.
There is nothing else I can eat.
Genetics – this isn't my fault.
Having a cheat meal/day will help me stay on track with the diet later.
I'll work out more later.
I'll just have a little bit.
In many cultures, being overweight is beautiful.
I'm too old.
This holiday wouldn't be special without eating this.
I don't have the ingredients I need.
I don't see any other choice here.
My family won't eat this.
I'm too stressed out.
I just worked out, so I can have this.
I'm going to go work out, so I can have this.
I'm too busy to deal with this today.

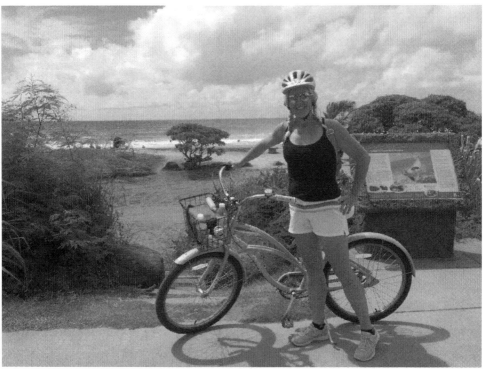

"Cheating" tastes great in the moment, but afterward, I am so regretful and angry at myself. I feel so much happier if I decide to do an "activity" instead.

I feel embarrassed about this.
I'll start again tomorrow.
I don't have time.
I'm not at my house right now.
I don't want to ask for special treatment.

None of these excuses are valid. Be honest with yourself here. A cheat meal might taste good in the moment, but will ultimately cause you stress and regret. Don't get mad now as you know I am right!

Loopholes aside, a cheat meal still counts as a cheat meal even if you didn't plan for it to happen. You can't blame your circumstances as a cause for failure. No matter if you are at a restaurant, at a relative's house, or even a work meeting, you are responsible for your choices. Do your research, speak up, and plan ahead.

What is more important to you, eating these "cheat meals" or being at a healthy weight with loads of energy? It's hard to see the forest through the trees at this point, I understand. If you have faith, however, I promise you, these small decisions will add up to a life more glorious than you have ever imagined.

THE BIG PICTURE

At this point, dear reader, I hope you are fired up to begin a DIRTY, LAZY, KETO diet. Armed with a keto shopping list and strong-willed, sassy attitude, you are now prepared to enter battle.

> *This mini-guide was meant to get you started down a new path, and now the follow through is in your hands.*

Like any war, there will be victories, and there will be set-backs. The scale might be your best friend on some days, worthy of tears of happiness, and even Instagram photos. You will revel in buying clothes in

113

smaller sizes and celebrate even the smallest private victories such as crossing your legs with ease. Now when I buckle my seatbelt on an airplane, I have the biggest smile on my face. It never gets old! Amusement park rides? YES, LET'S DO IT! I'm not worried about fitting inside of the safety bar or going over the weight limit. I feel like I'm finally living the life I was meant to live.

> *One of my fondest memories was the day my elementary school aged daughter wrapped her arms around me and yelled, "Mommy, my arms can reach completely around you!".*

Not every day will be full of sunshine and compliments, however, and I want you to plan for how you handle setbacks. Will you simply give up when the first roadblock presents itself, or will you rise to the occasion?

People often ask me what the hardest part was of losing 140 pounds. Was it running a marathon? *(I have finished twelve of them, thank you very much)*. Was it "coming back" after having eight body parts and a tumor surgically removed? (Nope, that wasn't it either, though that REALLY sucked!).

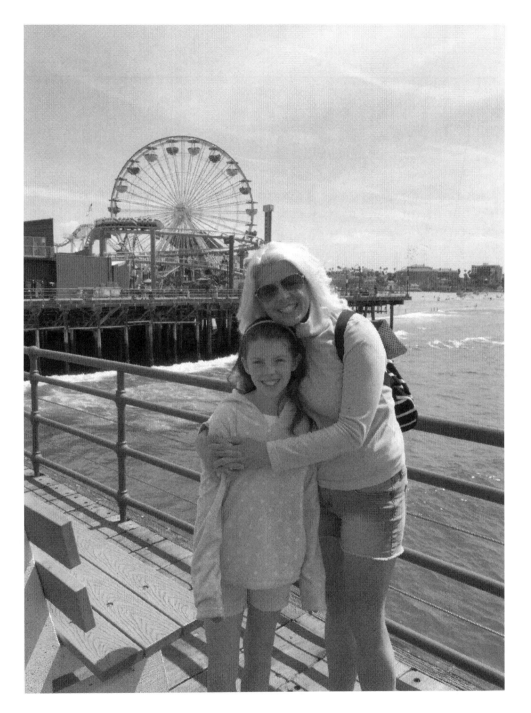

> *I'll tell you what the hardest part was... saying no to buttered popcorn at the movies. Yep, my answer is that simple.*

It's the little things that are the most challenging. **The little tiny decisions that we make all day long (that don't seem to matter) are actually what are most important**. These tiny decisions, over time, add up to huge lifestyle changes, and that is what DIRTY, LAZY, KETO is all about, my friends. This bit of advice (oh, and eating VEGETABLES!) is my personal secret sauce for long-term, sustainable, healthy weight loss.

You can do this, dear reader! Join me in the regular size section of the department store. Join me in the "normal" BMI category. Join me in ***putting yourself first***...

If I can lose half of my entire body weight and maintain the weight loss for more than five years, I'm betting with all of my heart that you can do this too.

See you on the other side...

Stephanie

XXOO

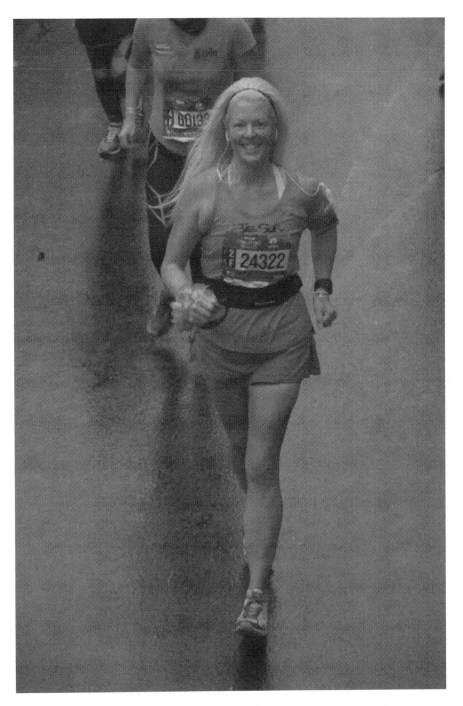

NEXT STEPS

Stay updated about the release of new mini-guides by registering your email at:
http://DirtyLazyKeto.com

Interact with the DIRTY, LAZY, KETO community by joining the author-led Facebook group:
https://www.facebook.com/groups/177473472816901

For continued support, new ideas, and inspiration, follow my frequent updates on social media at:

https://twitter.com/140lost
https://www.instagram.com/140lost/
https://www.facebook.com/140lost

RESOURCES

The following resources are recommended to help support your DIRTY, LAZY, KETO journey.

Books:

The Obesity Guide by Dr. Jason Fung, 2016
The Four Tendencies by Gretchen Rubin, 2018
The Case Against Sugar, by Gary Taubes, 2016
Why We Get Fat: And What to Do About It by Gary Taubes, 2011

Apps:

Carb Manager
MyFitnessPal
Fitbit
Yummly

Made in the USA
Lexington, KY
17 August 2019